"Our 'mysterious brain' enables us to perceive, think, feel, and behave, so it is vitally important that we keep it fit. BrainFit for Life uses neuroscience advances to promote our own brain health. As Executive Director of the first Comprehensive Depression Center in the world, I doubt any topic could be more important. Enjoy!"

John F. Greden, MD
Executive Director, University of Michigan,
Comprehensive Depression Center

"BrainFit For Life is vital for everything from daily living and work related success to long term happiness and health. This book supplies the tools needed to improve brain efficiency for a better, more focused and 'sharper' life experience. BrainFit For Life is a must for any lifelong total fitness plan."

Georgeanne Fayrweather
Triathlete and Fitness Professional

"We must change our thinking from cure to prevention. BrainFit For Life will not just demand your attention, it will give you the daily, all important game plan for change. This book is a must for kids from 1 to 100."

Dr. Dean Miller
Former NASA Director of Physiological Research

"BrainFit For Life is a hoot. The book details how the body and the brain must function together to make a person's life joyful. It will leave you chuckling and determined to try harder to do the right thing. There are no sermons, just a serenade on how beautiful life can be."

Jay Carp
Award Winning Author and Publisher

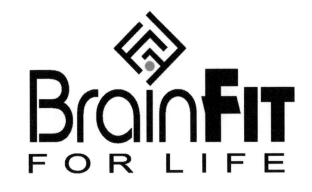

A User's Guide to Life-Long Brain Health and Fitness

by
Simon J. Evans, PhD
and Paul R. Burghardt, PhD

Published in the USA by
River Pointe Publications
Milan, Michigan 48160

Cataloging-in-Publication

Evans, Simon J. (Simon John), 1966-
  Brainfit for life : a user's guide to life-long brain health and fitness / by Simon J. Evans and Paul R. Burghardt.
       p. cm.
  Includes index.
  ISBN 978-0-9817258-0-2 (pbk.)
1. Brain--Diseases--Prevention--Popular works. 2. Brain--Aging--Prevention--Popular works. 3. Self-care, Health. I. Burghardt, Paul R. (Paul Ryen), 1976- II. Title.
  RC386.2.E93 2008
  613--dc22

                                        2008036805

Printed in the USA by McNaughton & Gunn

Note to Readers

This information and advice published or made available through the *BrainFit For Life*™ program is not intended to replace the services of a physician, nor does it constitute a doctor-patient relationship. Information in this book and on our web site is provided for informational purposes only and is not a substitute for professional medical advice. You should not use the information from this program for diagnosing or treating a medical or health condition. You should consult a physician in all matters relating to your health, and particularly in respect to any symptoms that may require diagnosis or medical attention. Any action on your part in response to the information provided in this book is at the reader's discretion. Readers should consult their own physicians concerning the information contained in this program. *BrainFit For Life*™ makes no representations or warranties with respect to any information offered or provided on or through the program materials regarding treatment, action, or application of medication. *BrainFit For Life*™ is not liable for any direct or indirect claim, loss or damage resulting from use of this book or any web sites linked from it.

Dedication

To my parents, Reg and Betty, who taught me to think. To my wife, Marne, who supports me even when I don't. And to my children, Aidan and Kian, who teach me not to think too much.

Simon

To my parents, Ann and Jon, and siblings, Jill, Jody, and Kyle for your loving support. To my wife Amy for her love, patience, and dedication. To my son, Evan for his love and inspiration.

Paul

Table of Contents

PREFACE

"If the brain were so simple we could understand it, we would be so simple we couldn't."

- Lyall Watson (author and anthropologist)

Why Did We Write *BrainFit For Life*?

We are neuroscientists. We love to try to figure out how the brain works and does all the cool stuff that it does. We also understand (referring to the above quote) that will probably never completely happen. However, brain science has made significant progress with some findings that can help us all take care of, and even improve, that big squishy organ between our ears. We know a lot about how the brain responds to all the daily stuff we do to it, what stuff makes it better and what stuff to avoid. We also both have a passion for healthy living. We're not total freaks about it. We planned some parts of this book over micro-brewed beers, other parts over coffee, or our favorite greasy sub sandwiches. We know the value of enjoying life through variety and moderation.

We see so much cool data coming out of the scientific community in regards to the role that healthy living plays in the health of your brain, but unfortunately, much of that information doesn't reach the public in any readable way. We scientists have our own language. We love to make up acronyms and use big, long words that sometimes seem like their sole purpose is to create confusion. Even scientists from slightly different fields can't understand each other half the time. So a major goal in writing this book is to translate some of the cool studies, coming from the field of brain research, into everyday conversational language. We must admit however, that we still like to make up acronyms and hope that you find some of them entertaining.

A bigger driver for writing this book is to be a small voice in promoting healthy living now, so that you can experience a bigger, stronger and faster brain as you age. Everyone knows that the lifestyle factors you choose have an effect on your health. But most people just think of their heart health. We are here to tell you that many of those same decisions have an effect on your brain as well. And we're not just talking about losing your mind as you age, but your brain performance today. Unfortunately, the behaviors so many people indulge in more and more in today's world are not setting them up for a bright mental future. This applies to kids, middle aged, and older adults. We want to raise awareness of the factors that help you create that future of keeping your *BrainFit For Life*.

Why Is This Important?

We know that we're living longer, but the question remains, are we living better? Mental illness accounts for the greatest socio-economic burden according to the World Health Organization. Currently 4.5 million individuals suffer from Alzheimer's disease. Due to an aging baby-boomer population, this number is expected to jump to 16 million by 2020 in the United States alone. Additionally, depression and anxiety disorders account for one of the largest burdens on quality of life for patients and loved ones. Finally, the rates of diabetes, heart disease and obesity are staggering and beginning to gain a foothold in children. There are currently no 'treatments' that cure or reverse the process of these diseases.

There is hope, but what do we need to do? First, we should realize that we are always fighting against convenience. We have easy food, easy transportation, easy entertainment, and we have a glut of it. However, if you are aware of your behavior you can gain control over how these conveniences affect your brain and body. And if you make the right choices the fruits of your efforts will be improved health and quality of life. That isn't to say this will all be easy. In fact, it may be quite difficult in some cases, but we want to help you succeed. It's part of the journey through life. As the Chinese proverb goes, *"A journey of a thousand miles begins with a single step."*

The brain is the final frontier. Many scientists consider it to be more complex than the rest of the known universe. It has about 100 billion neurons (brain cells), and it's estimated that on average each neuron makes 10,000 connections. This means you have about 10 trillion connections in your brain! As you read *BrainFit For Life*, much will happen in your brain. You will feel the texture of the pages, experience the smell of the book, see the contrast between ink and page, recognize the shapes that form letters, the patterns that create words and sentences, understand how the sentences and paragraphs convey information and conjure up images, and associate those images with personal meaning and value. These are the sensations that wire themselves into your brain and turn into lasting memories. Your brain is your portal for your perception of the physical world that you exist in, for better or worse. At the same time your brain provides you with the capability to remove yourself from your reality and create or experience worlds that are completely unique to each individual. Our brains are critically important to everything. It is what makes us human, it is what makes you, you. So now is the time to get your brain in shape, to make it *BrainFit For Life*!

Who Should Read *BrainFit For Life*?

We realize that the content of this book will be mainly attractive to older adults who may be starting to notice the effects of aging on their cognitive function. However, we hope that parents of school age kids will also take interest in this subject matter because the actions you and your kids take today truly have an impact on the grace with which you and they will age. It's difficult to think of your kids or grandkids as older adults, but that is who they will become and the more you help them out now the easier time they will have in their golden years.

Many of the approaches to incorporate brain fitness strategies into your lives are not age specific. In some cases they are best applied differently in an age-appropriate manner and we point that out throughout the text when this is the case.

We sincerely hope that you enjoy the content within the following pages and find inspiration to incorporate at least some of it into the habits of your life. You have control over your future and the future of your younger generations. This book is about empowering yourself and your family to enjoy life to its fullest. Be the example by living the best life you can.

Laying The Foundation

CHAPTER 1

INTRODUCTION TO BRAIN FITNESS

"The greatest discovery of my generation is that man can alter his life simply by altering his attitude of mind."
- William James, circa 1900 (psychologist and philosopher)

Your brain is changing and it will continue to change during your entire life. Yes, your brain is aging along with the rest of your body, but that's not all that we are talking about here. A very important thing to realize is that your brain responds and adapts to the environment you live in and the experiences that you have.

Whether you are asleep or awake, your brain is active. For example, your brain is busy taking care of all the stuff that you don't think about – like your heart rate, blood pressure and breathing. It's communicating with your digestive system and fat stores. It's talking to your immune system. Even when you are at rest, your brain acts very differently compared to other organs in your body.

If you're moving around, your brain is controlling your muscles, coordinating them to allow you to walk, run or hold this book. Your brain is also thinking, processing the words on this page, putting them into context based on your past experiences, so that you can understand them. While you are sleeping, your brain is busy restocking stores of brain chemicals in preparation for when you wake up. It is also controlling a surge of hormones throughout your body, resetting your internal clocks. It is busy replaying the experiences of the previous day, burning the memories into brain circuits for later recall and use.

Your brain is busy – and just the nature of all these activities is actually changing your brain. Just think! Thoughts are things. They are electrical and chemical activities that by their very existence are changing the physical structure of your brain. Although you can't stop all these modifications (and you wouldn't want to), you can have some control over them. The question then becomes, *are you changing your brain for better or for worse?*

Your brain is the master integrator of everything that you do, think and feel. Different parts of your brain talk to each other to exert control over your behavior, emotions, much of your metabolism, and your intellectual skills. Just like the rest of your body, your brain can be fit, and 'in shape', or unfit, and 'out of shape'. You can exercise your brain to improve your level of brain fitness.

However, like the rest of your body, it takes a variety of different workout routines to get your brain in great shape. If you went to the gym and did nothing but arm curls, your biceps would get strong but you wouldn't expect to improve the tone of your legs. To get a full body workout you need a mix of resistance training and aerobic activity on a regular basis. Improving your brain fitness works the same way. It takes a variety of approaches that we'll cover throughout this book.

How Long Is Your Brainspan?

We are fortunate enough today to expect to live about 20 years longer than our grandparents did. Since the 1950s, we have enjoyed a two-decade increase in lifespan. The downside is that there is a big difference between lifespan and healthspan, which is the number of years that you remain healthy. Although most people are living longer, it is an unfortunate reality that many are just dying more slower. A specific component of healthspan that most people care deeply about is their brainspan, or the number of years you maintain a healthy brain. Alzheimer's disease and other types of dementia are probably the most feared diseases. Often times dementia goes hand in hand with depression and metabolic problems, such as obesity or heart disease, as well. The vast majority of people rank brain health at the top of their list for quality of life indicators. The more fit your brain, the better and happier you feel.

Over the age of 65, there is a 5% chance of developing Alzheimer's disease. Over the age of 85, those odds jump to 50%. But frankly, those statistics are much scarier than they need to be. When people hear statistics like that, they tend to feel helpless, as if they are rolling the dice. However, when it comes to your brainspan you can weigh the dice in your favor. This book is a guide to help you weigh the dice and dramatically reduce your odds of ending up on the dark side of statistics. We want to help you remain *BrainFit For Life*.

Saying that people over 85 have a 50% chance of having Alzheimer's disease is a little misleading. The real statement is that by the age of 85, 50% of people have Alzheimer's disease. That may seem like the same thing, but it's really a very different statement. Putting it the first way, it seems that everyone has a 50-50 chance of getting Alzheimer's disease, but that's not really true. Some folks have a very high chance, while others are completely safe. *Your* chance of developing Alzheimer's by the age of 85 is not necessarily 50% – so what is it? We want you to know that there are many things you can do to improve the odds of developing and keeping your brain healthy, and that's what this book is about.

Here, we use Alzheimer's disease as one specific example, but we will discuss your ability to improve your odds of maintaining life-long brain fitness from a number of different perspectives.

Factors like diet, exercise, sleep habits, and the degree to which you workout your brain all play a significant role. There are also other factors that are mostly outside your control (although not completely unchangeable). For example, your genes certainly play some role in your brain fitness, but you even have some control over those. See the *Neural Nugget #1, A New Pair of Genes*, following this introduction for a look at how you influence your genetic makeup. The environment in which you've spent your life so far is past your control. Even if it was not ideal, you can't go back and change it. But you can change any part of your environment going forward. The remaining chapters will focus on many of the factors that control your odds of keeping your brain fit. We'll attend to all of these in the sections to follow.

EPIC Performance

You may have already heard the term brain fitness thrown around before. A lot of effort is currently going into providing intellectually challenging software games in an attempt to help the mind stay young. While this is one important factor, this book is about boosting *total* brain fitness, which we break down into three main cognitive systems. Before going any further, we'll tell you what we mean by 'cognition'. There are many definitions for this term, but we'll stick with Webster's, which is "the act of knowing, knowledge, or perception". We will discuss Emotional, Physical and Intellectual Cognition, what we call your EPIC performance. Let's take a little deeper look at what these are:

1. <u>Emotional Intelligence (EQ)</u>. Your brain controls your mood and your ability to handle stress and respond to challenges. It controls your ability to read the emotions of others and respond appropriately. Your emotional intelligence, or EQ, is the aspect of brain fitness that has a large impact on your self confidence, day to day mood and success in social environments, including career and family life. For the most part, a system in your brain called your cortico-limbic system is responsible for controlling your emotional intelligence, and like most systems in your brain, you can improve it with specific focus.

2. <u>Physical intelligence (PQ)</u>. Your brain also controls much of the rest of your body, but it is important to recognize that this is a two-way street. There is a constant conversation between your brain and your heart, your lungs, your digestive system, your immune system and many other parts of your physiology. Your brain is 'listening' to other parts of your body by monitoring hormones and signals put out by those organs. It responds to those signals with instructions that, in turn, control the activity of your organs. Your physical intelligence, or PQ, controls how successfully you maintain your weight and cardiovascular health; effectively handle illness with your immune response; and physically respond to stress. A major player in all of this is a part of your brain called the hypothalamus. The daily actions you choose also control this aspect of brain fitness.

3. <u>Intellectual Cognition (IQ)</u>. Finally, your brain controls your ability to learn and remember things, solve problems, make decisions and act creatively. Your intellectual cognition affects your success in school, business and your

career. Furthermore, your ability to maintain your intellectual cognition determines your quality of life, especially in your golden years. Intellectual brain fitness is most reliant on the outer part of your brain, called your cortex, but it also relies on regions underneath your cortex, called your thalamus and hippocampus. Because of the incredibly flexible nature of these particular brain regions, your actions greatly influence the fitness level of these brain circuits.

Although we separate out these functions and brain systems for ease of discussion, you must realize that they are all related. Because of that, focusing on one brain healthy behavior will have carry-over benefit to the others. Focusing on several brain healthy behaviors will provide a synergistic effect to propel you forward. We'll discuss how you can use multiple approaches at the same time, to your best advantage.

The Four Cornerstones Of Brain Fitness

You can work on every component of your EPIC performance discussed above, with focus on the four cornerstones of brain fitness, which are:

1. Quality Nutrition. What you choose to put in your mouth becomes the raw materials for building and maintaining brain circuits. Foods and supplements can dramatically affect the way your entire brain works. Science has shown us that various nutrients affect brain circuits that control mood, metabolism and intellectual abilities. Section 1 details how nutrition affects your emotional, physical and intellectual cognition and identifies some nutrients to consider getting into your regular routine.

2. <u>Physical activity</u>. Exercise is probably the closest thing that we have to a fountain of youth. Study after study has shown that physical activity in kids and adults of all ages improves brain function on many levels. It helps you regulate stress, boosts your metabolism, improves your ability to learn and remember, and improves your performance on various types of cognitive tests. Section 2 outlines what we know about how exercise helps your brain on all aspects of your EPIC performance and provides you with fun, age appropriate guidelines to help you get physical activity into your life.

3. <u>Mental activity</u>. Like anything else, your brain follows the 'use it or lose it' rule. You will strengthen the brain circuits that get regular use. Likewise, if you stop using certain brain circuits, they will wither and fade. Some very cool studies over the last several years show benefits of life-long learning in reducing Alzheimer's disease and other types of cognitive decline. Section 3 discusses how staying engaged in life contributes to your overall brain fitness and provides some plans on how to ensure enough variety in your life to maximize this benefit.

4. <u>Sleep</u>. Getting enough downtime is as important as getting enough activity. Although it may seem like time lost, sleep is a critically active period for your brain. It is a time when you restock important brain chemicals, consolidate memories and regulate an army of hormones that control your metabolism. Each person requires a certain amount of sleep to allow their brain to complete these vital tasks. Section 4 details the importance of sleep and rest for creating and maintaining life-long brain health with some specific plans to get you there.

Think of the four cornerstones of brain fitness like the four legs of a table. If all four legs are loose, the table may still look fine and remain standing. However, when you stress the table by putting a heavy object on it, it will likely collapse. Tightening just one leg of the table will have carry over benefit to the stability of the entire surface. But the table will still remain vulnerable to collapse if you stress it with a heavy object over an unstable leg. Any weak leg will compromise the strength of the entire table.

When you work on the four cornerstones of brain fitness, you tighten all four legs of the table. Then it doesn't matter where the stress comes from. You could place a heavy object anywhere on the table and it would remain stable. Similarly, when you focus on all aspects of brain fitness you can more easily handle day-to-day stress in your life or the stress of aging or disease and remain strong and stable.

The cool thing is that you can work on brain fitness at any age. Like anything else, the sooner you start the better, but it is never too late for some improvement. That is why we hope that all generations will take these messages to heart. We understand that older adults may have the most personal concern about brain fitness. But we hope that parents of school age kids take notice for themselves and their children as well because today's actions determine tomorrow's results.

The Inverted U

I'm sure you've heard the statement that if something is good then more must be better. Hopefully, you realize that this is only true to a point. There is a concept in science called the 'inverted U', which applies to almost everything in nature, including us. It's a concept represented by an upside down U, or inverted U, as we science geeks call it. It simply shows that more of anything causes an effect to a point, and then it either stops having an affect or begins to have an opposite effect. The easiest way to represent this is using a graph. We are scientists and scientists love graphs. Instead of explaining something to us, we'd rather just look at the graph. We make graphs, we read graphs, we interpret graphs, we dream about graphs and we eat graphs for breakfast. We realize that most readers don't share our love of graphs and we promise not to load this book with them. But we have to include this very simple one to make this point because it is a point that will re-emerge many times throughout the following chapters. Looking at the graph below, you see an upside down U shaped curve.

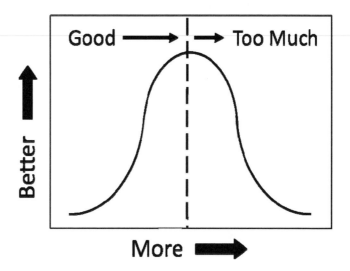

This simple representation just says that more is not always better. Everything has an optimum. Pharmacologists use this principle all the time in drug design studies to find the concentration of a drug that has the best effect. Weight lifters use it to find the right weight to build muscle without ripping themselves to shreds. Teachers use it to give their students the right amount of information that will encourage new thinking without overloading their students' brains. Even Goldilocks used it to find the porridge that was just the right temperature; not too hot and not too cold. You will also see us use it when talking about the four cornerstones of brain fitness.

Returning to our table analogy, when you get all of the legs of your table tightened up just right, you have a very strong surface. But what if you were a little over-zealous in tightening one of the legs and you stripped the screw or broke the bolt? That wouldn't be good. Whether we're talking about nutrition, exercise, mental workouts or sleep, there is an optimal point that will do you the most good. But here's the next point. Everyone's optimal point is different. There is no perfect diet for everyone. Your physical workout routine might kill your neighbor. Your mental workout routine might make someone else's head explode. The amount of sleep you need may not be the same as your spouse or your boss, and certainly not your kids.

Because this is true, we are not going to give you a perfect diet and exercise plan. We're not going to tell you that the magic formula for mental clarity is 12 crossword puzzles, 5 Sudokus and a jumble every week. We can't tell you exactly how much sleep you need. What we will do, is give you an understanding of the basic principles that will help you design your own optimal plan. Importantly, it's not just about stuff that's good for you, but also the stuff you like, you can afford and you have access to. We make every attempt throughout this book to keep it practical, while at the same time backing it up with science. Don't worry, we're not going to 'data dump' on you either, but we will give you some cool studies that highlight the main points. If you want to dig deeper into any topic we discuss, you can refer to the resource section in the back of this book or visit BrainFitForLife.com/resources for updates.

How Is This Book Organized?

We organized this book into four main sections. Each section is devoted to one of the cornerstones of brain fitness. At the end of the book, we'll conclude with a discussion about methods to improve your global level of cognitive health and action plans to achieve it. We understand that some people will pick up a book and read it from cover to cover in the order printed. Other people just want to pick out a few pieces of specific information that they are looking for. We have written this book to accommodate both types of readers. The book flows in a logical sequence to help you understand all the factors associated with boosting your level of brain fitness, including action plans at the end of each section. At the same time, the sections are self-contained so that you can quickly find complete information specific to each subtopic. Additionally, we have inserted '*Neural Nuggets*' in between some of the chapters to provide a little deeper discussion on some key parts of brain fitness.

We promise you that by the end of this book you will have a better appreciation of all the stuff you are doing on a daily basis to change your brain. We hope that by the end of this book that stuff will be changing your brain for the better.

On your mark. Get set. Go.

Neural Nugget #1 – A New Pair Of Genes

What Do Your Genes Have To Do With It?

Genetics certainly play a role in the grace with which you age, but there is much more to the story. Many studies show that lifestyle choices dramatically affect your odds of staying healthy. In other words, you have control over what your odds are, and that is good news.

In this day and age, everyone has heard of genetics and has some idea what that term means. But we need to take a minute to explain some things just a little deeper in order to give you an understanding of how much control you have over your genes.

First of all, let's talk briefly about what a gene is. It's really just a blueprint. Genes themselves don't do that much. The proteins built from the instructions in the genes are what do most of the work. Think of a gene as the instructions for building a machine, like a car, washing machine, or hair-dryer. Each of these does a specific job. Cars get you from point A to point B, washing machines clean your clothes and hair dryers dry your hair. Yet, there are many different models and varieties of each of these. Some cars get better gas mileage. Some washing machines handle bigger loads. Some hair dryers have more power.

Genes are similar in that they code for proteins that have specific jobs to do in our cells, but they come in different models and that's what makes us different. We all have the types of genes (20,000 or so by estimates at the time of this writing), but many of them come in different varieties. For example, we all have a gene that codes for the pigment in our eye, but the make and model of that gene is what determines our eye color. On a more physiological basis, we all have a gene for hemoglobin that transports oxygen through our blood, but some models are more efficient at delivering oxygen than others. Scientists refer to different models, or gene varieties, as alleles (a-leels). Some genes only have one known allele and so we all have exactly the same model for that gene. Other genes have two or more alleles. Multiply all the different alleles by the number of different genes and that leads to genetic variation among people.

To go a little further, genes rarely work alone. For example there is no gene for height, shoe size, or ability to run a 4-minute mile, but there are sets of genes that all contribute to these physical attributes. You inherit genes from your parents. So you don't have any control over the various gene alleles or models that you have.

But that's not the end of the story; there is another component to genetics that you do have control over. Before you can build the proteins, that get together to do their jobs, the genes that code for those proteins must be active. You can't drive the blueprints for a car. First, a factory crew must build the car. Furthermore, depending on how many cars you need, the factory crew could build a large number from just one set of instructions. Genes can also output many copies of their coded protein, depending on how active the genes are. Scientists refer to the activity level of genes as gene expression. The more highly a gene is expressed, the more copies of the protein, and the more work those proteins can do, and this is something that you have a great deal of control over.

Some genes are important to all of your cells and are active all the time. For example, the genes that code for proteins that build the physical scaffolding or the framework of your cells are highly expressed in all cells. Other genes are very specialized and are only expressed in specific cell types. To use hemoglobin again, it is highly expressed in red blood cells but not really in anything else because it's the red blood cells job to carry oxygen around the body.

Nearly all the cells in your body have two copies of every single gene. But different cell types, like brain cells, heart cells and blood cells have different specialized functions so they express different sets of genes. They only activate the genes required for the job those cells need to do.

Why the long-winded explanation? Because you need to realize you have a lot of control over gene expression. The foods you eat, the activities you do and the stress you feel all have a huge impact on gene expression. This is the part of your genetics that you can control. Even though you are stuck with the genes you inherited from your folks, you can influence how they get used.

Before we leave this topic, there's one more piece to the genetic puzzle that you should be aware of. This is getting into an area of science that we are really just beginning to unravel, called epigenetics (literally meaning 'outside of genetics'). Sometimes when you activate or inactivate a gene it is a very short-term effect. For example, a bout of exercise will crank up some genes that protect your cells from oxygen damage. Other times a chronic behavior can have a long-term effect on your genes by actually modifying them in a way to permanently increase or decrease their expression. This is called 'imprinting'. Not all genes can be imprinted, but those that can, tend to play significant roles in maintaining your physiology.

The surprising thing that we are learning now, is that these modifications can be passed down to future generations. This is especially true during pregnancy. We all know that a mother's diet, stress levels and other lifestyle factors can have an effect on the development of the baby-to-be. Interestingly, part of this effect is through imprinting genes to permanently crank them up or tune them down.

From a developmental perspective, this makes a lot of sense. Essentially the mother is fore-warning her baby as to what kind of environment he or she will be born into. If the mother is low on nutrients during pregnancy, the baby interprets that as not having a lot of food in the environment, so will turn up genes required for energy storage. This is great preparation if indeed the baby will be born into an environment with a lack of food. However, if the mother is just eating poorly and the baby is actually born into an environment with plenty of food, they will now have the disadvantage of storing energy too efficiently and potentially face a life-long struggle against obesity.

The surprising thing that we are learning is that imprinting can be passed down through multiple generations from either the father or the mother. The lifestyle you choose to live has an effect on how your genes are imprinted and this modification can be stable through your kids' lives and sometimes passed onto their kids as well. Applying the four cornerstones of brain fitness that we will discuss throughout the rest of this book will help you optimize gene expression to improve and maintain your brain health for yourself, and potentially your offspring. If you are done with the procreation part of your life, you can still influence the brain fitness of future generations through the habits that you instill in your children and grandchildren today.

The First Cornerstone

Quality Nutrition

CHAPTER 2

BRAIN MATTER MATTERS
Introduction To Nutritional Approaches For Brain Fitness

"To eat is a necessity, but to eat intelligently is an art."
- Francois La Rochefoucauld, circa 1650 (author)

Nutrition is a key part of any health plan, including cognitive fitness. Whatever you decide to allow past your lips, into your mouth and down to your gut becomes the raw materials used to build brain circuits and body tissues. Some of those materials will support productive growth and maintenance. Others will tip the scales toward decline and degeneration. So it goes well beyond the phrase, "What goes past the lips heads straight for the hips;" it also gets to the brain.

Your brain is full of very powerful hormones and other 'signaling' molecules, which have a huge effect on your mood and cognitive abilities. When you trace the origins of where these all come from, you eventually get back to your diet. Many components of food are 'neuroactive', meaning that they can directly stimulate or inhibit brain cell activity. Other components of your diet influence how these neuroactive compounds work, and still others act as the raw materials for producing them. All of these diet-derived neuroactive molecules have dramatic influences on the way you feel, the clarity with which you think, the way you behave in response to other people, the way you handle stress, and the way that your brain controls the rest of your body. Your diet literally influences your thoughts and emotions. The old adage 'you are what you eat' applies to your brain as well.

Your body is incredibly good at breaking foods down into their basic building blocks and putting them back together into what you need. However, your body cannot make many of the nutrients it needs. This defines the *essential* vitamins, minerals, amino acids and fats. These are building blocks required for the construction of our brain and body cells, which we must get from our diets or in supplement form. In this section, we will discuss the role of some fundamental concepts and key nutrients for optimizing your emotional, physical and intellectual fitness, your EPIC performance.

This section is not about providing you with a specific diet. There are plenty of books out there for that. Besides, there is no perfect diet for everyone. Some things will work well for you and not well for others. We are all genetically diverse and have different physiologies. We also have different likes and dislikes, which contribute substantially to whether or not you will adhere to any given diet plan.

Instead, our goal is to provide you with fundamental concepts that you can apply to any diet you choose. To be clear, by diet, we mean a *sustainable lifestyle approach* to eating. Although, there are short-term approaches that can be useful to set up your metabolism for longer term success, you should always view these in the context of long-term lifestyle approaches. We will give you a basic understanding of how different nutrients contribute to the way your brain and body functions, and this will help you find the right plan you will enjoy and will work for you. Later in the section, we will get into some specific nutrients that science has shown to be beneficial for brain function and some food sources where you can get them.

The good news about nutritional affects on your brain is that your brain is very selective about which nutrients it allows in. You have a special 'guard wall' called the blood-brain barrier. This barrier carries on a constant vigil to protect your brain by keeping stuff it doesn't want on the outside, and stuff it needs on the inside. Furthermore, your brain usually gets first dibs on the essential nutrients, so it will often be the last organ to experience deficiency. However, this guard wall is not perfect. Some toxic substances can escape detection and get in; and if you don't get enough essential nutrients into your diet, your brain will eventually become deficient in the good stuff as well. You may initially notice nutrient deficiencies as fatigue, feelings of irritation or a general lack of clear thinking. If you allow deficiency to continue, you may experience more substantial and chronic signs of physical and cognitive decline. We'll talk about what you can do to avoid that throughout this section.

Turning Food Into Energy

Beyond getting first dibs on nutrients, your brain is also an energy hog. Your brain claims about 20% of your food energy, even though it totals about 2% of your bodyweight. So it demands 10 times its share by weight. Brain cells are packed with little power plants, called mitochondria. These do the majority of the work in creating useful energy. Think of them like a refinery, where the broken down food turns into the fuel of choice for most of the cell's operations (a molecule called ATP). But a cost of producing a lot of energy is the potential for damage from toxic by-products of the production process, and this can lead to a process called oxidative stress.

We're not going to go into a lot of technical detail, but this is a major concept that you should be aware of because oxidative stress potentially underlies many different chronic degenerative diseases, including some cases of Alzheimer's disease and other cognitive disorders. Essentially, the foods and nutrients you eat can have a huge impact in terms of promoting oxidative stress or protecting you from it, and this in turn increases or decreases your risk of disease.

Typically, toxic by-products from energy production are kept under control, but every once in a while there is a leak in the system and a 'free radical' escapes. A free radical is a very unstable molecule that is looking to steal (an electron) from something else in order to become stable again. When this happens, it can lead to the destructive process of oxidative stress. Oxygen is a double edged sword, we need it for energy production, but its reactivity can make it very dangerous.

The problem is that whatever molecular victim the free radical steals an electron from, has to go steal an electron from another molecule to return itself to a stable state. It's kind of like a game of tag-you're-it. However, instead of the molecules just tagging each other they rip off a piece of the other's skin and damage it. This can cause a chain reaction of electron stealing that can potentially damage genes or important proteins.

Since the brain is a big user and producer of energy, it must be especially vigilant to keep oxidative stress under control. You can help your brain do this in a couple of ways. First, eat foods that will not create too much oxidative stress, which we'll cover later. Second, get plenty of nutrients that protect against oxidative stress. It's a no-brainer really. Keep the bad foods out of your diet (because they foster oxidative stress) and get the good foods in (because they help keep oxidative stress under control). As you increase the ratio of good food to bad food, you will gain control over the levels of oxidative stress in your brain and body.

Many years of poor dieting can lead to an accumulation of damage from oxidative stress and eventually lead to disease. You're not going to develop major damage after one poor meal choice, but continued poor choices over the years can be problematic. It just depends on where the damage happens as

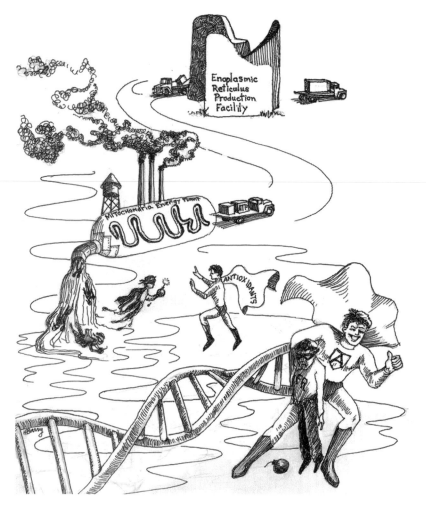

"The antioxidant super heroes stand guard over the mitochondrial energy production plants to capture escaping free radical villains before they can do damage to your cell.".

to whether or not disease develops, and what the disease looks like. This is where your genes can come into play as well. Oxidative stress can be most damaging wherever you are genetically weakest. If you have a family history of a certain illness then you likely have a genetic predisposition toward that illness. A poor diet, through oxidative stress, is one thing that can push you down that road faster. Too much oxidative damage in the brain seems to underlie some cases of Alzheimer's, Parkinson's and other neurodegenerative diseases. Likewise, eating quality foods that protect against oxidative stress can help you stave off disease, even if you have a genetic predisposition toward it. Your diet can protect you from, or propel you down your genetic path.

In the remainder of this chapter, we'll discuss what types of foods help you accomplish optimal brain fitness. Then, in the next few chapters we'll get into some specifics regarding how your diet contributes to your emotional, physical and intellectual health. We'll start the discussion by breaking nutrients into the major categories of macronutrients and micronutrients. However, understand that these two classes of nutrients depend on each other. We only separate them here for simplicity of the discussion.

Macronutrients Provide Balance For Your Brain

Macronutrients (as the name implies) are big nutrients. These are your proteins, carbohydrates and fats that you may have read about in any diet book. Your body requires some of each of these in order to build new cells for your brain and body. Proteins help build strength, structure and stability in our cells. Carbohydrates provide us with the energy we need, and yes, fat can be good for us as well. One fact that surprises many people is that your brain is actually about 65% fat! Your brain is one big fatty organ. However, it needs the right kind of fat for optimal function.

Fat Is Good . . . Sometimes

Although the media has done a good job at brainwashing many folks into believing that fat is bad, this is a misleading message. Fats serve many essential functions, especially in the brain. On the whole-body scale, fat helps insulate and protect all your major organs. On the microscopic scale, a layer of fat surrounds every one of your cells to form the membrane that keeps the inside separated from the outside of the cell. Neurons (brain cells) have huge amounts of membranes because of their complexity, so they require a lot of fat.

But fats come in many forms. They can be saturated, mono-unsaturated or poly-unsaturated. You need them all. However, even though we need saturated fat, your body can make just about all that it needs and most people get way more than is needed in their diet. Also, saturated fat is more easily oxidized and contributes to oxidative stress. That's one reason why too much saturated fat is associated with heart disease and why you should try to minimize the saturated fat in the foods that you eat.

On the other hand, mono-unsaturated and poly-unsaturated fats are healthy for the brain and the heart. It's more difficult for our bodies to make these and some forms can't be made at all, meaning we must get them from dietary sources. You'll find heart and brain-healthy monounsaturated fats at high concentrations in olive oil and other components of the touted 'Mediterranean diet'. Polyunsaturated fats include the much talked about omega-3s, and you'll find them in fish and some nuts and vegetables. Since omega-3s are crucial for overall brain health, we'll dig deeper into them and all the roles that they play in different aspects of brain fitness, in the *Neural Nugget #2, Fish Food*, at the end of this chapter.

Carbohydrates Are Brain Fuel

Carbohydrates are your main source of energy for your brain. In fact, the brain relies almost exclusively on energy derived from carbohydrates so you should consider them an important part of your brain-friendly diet. They are chains of sugars that are broken down and used to make the currency of your body's energy, a molecule called ATP. There is much disagreement among the diet gurus about how many carbohydrates to eat, ranging from about 40% to about 80% of your total calories. Frankly, different diet plans will work for different people but it is becoming clear that you should at least pay attention to the type of carbohydrates that you eat since not all carbohydrates are created equal.

Carbohydrates line up along the glycemic index scale, which is a measure of how fast your body breaks them down and releases them into the blood as sugar. The faster they spike your blood sugar, the higher the glycemic index number. The scale runs from 0 to 100, the high end of which is defined by 100% glucose (your brain relies exclusively on glucose for energy, but you want to provide it in a low-glycemic, 'slow-release' form). A high glycemic diet has been shown to increase markers of oxidative stress by cranking up the energy production machinery too quickly. So paying attention to this alone, will go a long way toward protecting yourself from this damaging process. Your body and your brain will perform much better if you eat carbohydrates that have a low glycemic index and raise your blood sugar slowly and steadily. These are mostly fruits, vegetables and whole grain products.

Imagine driving a car where you step on the gas as hard as you can and accelerate until you need to slam on the brakes to stop for a traffic light. Then as soon as you are through the light or stop sign, you accelerate as fast as possible until you need to slam on the brakes again for the next stop. Have you ever been in a car when the driver is driving like this? Contrast this to driving where you easily accelerate to get to a comfortable cruising speed before you easily decelerate when you need to stop. Although the first style may be exciting (for a while), which driving style is more stressful for you, your passengers, your engine and your brakes? Which driving style will keep the car in better running condition and get more miles out of it?

This is comparable to eating a low or a high glycemic diet. With a fast-burning carbohydrate-rich diet (high in sugar) you are continually spiking and crashing your energy production systems and creating stress for many of your biological systems, including your brain. Alternatively, a slow-burning, fiber-rich carbohydrate diet puts your energy producing systems into a steady mode, and reduces stress on your brain and body.

This is one reason why eating small meals frequently throughout the day, rather than big meals a few times a day, are much better for your health. Small meals will not pack a blood-sugar spiking punch and will help you maintain an even supply of energy. This is good for your brain, which needs that steady input, and also good for your metabolism, making it much easier to regulate your weight.

Interestingly, a recent study showed that timing is also important. It seems that we are much more susceptible to spiking our blood sugar in the morning than at later times in the day. This means that if you eat a high glycemic breakfast (like donuts, waffles, pancakes, sugared cereals, pastries, etc.) you will spike your blood sugar much higher than if you indulged in these foods around lunch or dinner. While we're not suggesting that you have donuts for lunch, if you absolutely can't give up the sweet stuff, you should at least try to avoid them in the morning meal. Having a breakfast higher in protein is one of the best things you can do to set your brain up for a productive day.

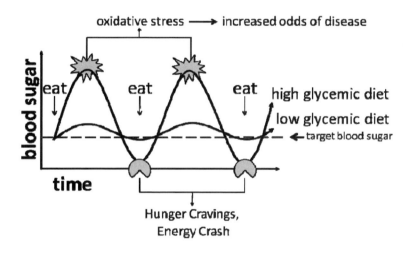

Proteins Get Stuff Done

Proteins are the major workhorses of your brain and body cells. They perform most of the jobs in the cell, moving things around and rearranging other molecules. In fact, proteins are the machinery used to make the needed fats and carbohydrates or to modify the ones we get from our diet. Proteins are long chains of amino acids that come in many shapes and sizes. They are responsible for carrying oxygen in your blood, contracting your muscles to allow you to move and transmitting messages through your brain circuits.

As discussed in the introduction, proteins are the products actually coded for in your genes. Each gene is a unique blueprint for a specific protein. We all have pretty much the same genes but have different variants of those genes and this is where genetic diversity and predisposition to health or disease comes into play.

Your body can make any protein it needs from the amino acid building blocks, but it can only make 12 of the 20 common amino acids building blocks from scratch. You must obtain the other 8 amino acids from your diet. So even though you make all the proteins you need by reading your genetic blueprint, you still have to eat proteins to get the essential amino acid building blocks. Even for the amino acids that you can make from scratch, it's much cheaper (energetically speaking) to eat them, than to make them.

Micronutrients Are The Unsung Heroes

The other major components of nutrition are micronutrients. These are typically much smaller than the macronutrients (although not always) and are the vitamins, minerals and other small molecule nutrients that your body needs for its daily duties. Today we know of 13 essential vitamins, meaning you cannot make these vitamins from scratch and have to get them from your diet. You must also obtain all of the minerals that you need from your diet. Some we require in large amounts, like Calcium, Sodium and Potassium. Others, called trace minerals, we require in smaller amounts, like Zinc, Copper and Manganese. A high quality multi-vitamin / multi-mineral can help you get all of these in the appropriate doses.

So what do micronutrients actually do? The answer to this question is the subject of volumes of text books, so again, rather than provide an entire thesis on nutrition, we'll stick to some basic concepts. In general, micronutrients are supporting actors in most of the hundreds of thousands of processes that go on in all of your cells, all of the time. While the macronutrients play the starring roles in your biochemistry, they wouldn't get much done without the micronutrients.

One major role that many micronutrients play is acting as antioxidants to help minimize oxidative damage and oxidative stress, which we previously discussed. Many vitamins have antioxidant properties to halt free radicals in their tracks. If you remember, free radicals sometimes escape from the energy production process to start a chain reaction of electron stealing that can cause damage. Antioxidants have extra electrons to donate to the free radicals so they never get started on their rampage through the cell.

It's very important to provide a variety of antioxidants so they are always available in different parts of your cells and tissues to halt oxidative stress. Some do a better job in fat tissue, others are better inside the water part of cells, and others do better floating around in the blood. This is why variety is key. In fact, the color of fruits and vegetables represents the type of vitamins and antioxidants they contain. If you strive to eat different colored fruits and vegetables every day you will help provide a variety of antioxidant protection.

Many foods, particularly unprocessed foods, contain all three macronutrients and many micronutrients, so they will contribute some portion of what our bodies need. However, you should try to be aware of what you are eating, even if you think you are eating 'healthy' or 'organic' because this doesn't necessarily mean you are getting a good balance of nutrients. Processed or refined foods are particularly tricky. They can be super-tasty, have a freakishly long shelf life, or be some incredible color never seen naturally on this planet. But in most cases they have had most of the nutritional value removed by the manufacturing process. Fortified processed foods can be especially misleading. Often times the food has most of the vitamins and minerals stripped out of them, then with a few of them added back earns the label, 'fortified'. Relying heavily on these sources of food can get you into trouble.

Vitamin Supplements – To Take Or Not To Take? That Is The Question.

The amount of essential vitamins needed is a matter of debate, but one measure is the RDA or Recommended Daily Allowance. The National Academy of Science first published the RDA in 1941 as the amount of specific vitamins and minerals required to prevent malnutrition. Back then, vitamin deficiencies that caused things like rickets and scurvy were not that uncommon. We needed a program to ensure that everyone got enough essential nutrients in their diets to keep them out of deficiency disease – so we created the RDA to do that. Overall, it has been very successful at its mission. You don't see too many people walking around with *severe* nutritional deficiencies any more (at least not in fortunate developed countries).

As our knowledge grew over time, we realized that RDA levels of micronutrients to avoid malnutrition were not the same as the levels needed for optimizing health. So in the 1990's the National Academy of Science introduced RDI (Reference Dietary Intakes), which are geared toward maintenance of optimal health. However, many nutritional experts have challenged even these as insufficient to promote optimal health throughout life, especially as record numbers of the population are reaching older years. The truth is that for many micronutrients, we don't really know what the optimal levels are and they are likely to be different for each individual person. Furthermore, what you need may change as you age. It will be somewhat dependent on the genes you inherited, your activity level and a whole host of other stuff that's really hard to measure. In many cases, the best we can do is to understand that the RDA levels represent a *minimum* amount of what we need on a daily basis.

It's unlikely that most people eating a typical western diet get all of the vitamins and minerals they need from their food. If you eat a very good diet, you can probably reach RDA levels, but probably not do much better than that for many essential nutrients. In fact a study from Yale, published in the late 1980s found that about 80% of people who felt they ate a good diet were not even meeting RDA levels for all the essential vitamins and minerals. That's not 80% of all people, but 80% of those who think they eat well, are still not getting even the minimum amount of nutrients.

Some people argue that we *should* be able to get everything we need from our food without taking nutritional supplements. After all, our ancestors never took supplements. They weren't introduced until about the 1940s. However, let's look a little deeper at some reasons that argue for supplementation.

First, the average cave-man (or woman) probably didn't live much past their twenties, so they didn't really have to worry about diseases of old-age. By the early 1900's, the average lifespan was still only in the fifties. Today, we are living much longer, which gives us far greater opportunity to accumulate damage from oxidative stress, so we would do well to start combating that stress earlier in life.

Second, the nutrient density of our ancestors' foods was much higher. Their foods were usually fresher, meaning the vitamin content was higher. As we harvest fruits and vegetables early, store them for longer periods and ship them across the country, the vitamin content goes down. Also, the mineral content in the soils has declined because we use the same land over and over again to grow our crops. Even though we put back some of the major minerals required for the plants to grow, these are not all the minerals required for life-long human health.

Third, our ancestors ate a lot less, so they didn't have as much food to process through the energy production channels. This means they probably also had less free radical production and oxidative stress. In fact, piles of studies from animal research show that if you feed them less, they live longer. This concept, called caloric-restriction, seems to work by cranking up genes that promote longevity, but also by minimizing damage from over active food processing.

Each of these provides reasons why today's environment can't be fairly compared to that of even 100 years ago. Times are different and a quality multi-vitamin / multi-mineral seems to be a good way to help maintain life-long health for your brain and your body. You can check our resource section for further advice on nutritional supplements.

Snake Oils To Watch Out For

Be wary of any single nutritional product that claims to fix everything from diabetes to dementia and depression. No food, juice, nutrition product or nutrient cures everything for everyone. Plenty of products out there claim to be everything you need to maintain your health. However, there is no magic bullet. Some of these products have a health benefit, but many are completely untested and unregulated, so buyer beware. You are best off eating a well balanced diet as discussed throughout this section and supplementing with a high quality science-based multi-vitamin/multi-mineral complex. Good nutrition product manufacturers use Good Manufacturing Practices, or

GMPs, which are universal standards of quality control that the FDA imposes on pharmaceutical companies. You can find some recommendations in the resources section at the back this book.

Another thing to be aware of is a new technology called nutrigenomics. This emerging field is a legitimate and exciting area of research, with promises to cater nutritional plans to your individual genes. We know something about a few of those gene-nutrient interactions already, as is the case for folate, which we discuss further in the next chapter. However, there is not nearly enough data yet to warrant spending your money on these nutrigenomic nutritional plans. We have a handle on the interaction between nutrition and a few dozen gene variants, but we have millions of gene variants yet to characterize. New genetic technologies are driving discovery in the nutrigenomics field, but it will be several years before it will be of value to the consumer, so you'd do well to keep your money in your pocket for now.

Moving On

With these basics in mind, you can move through the remaining chapters in this section, which get into the details of nutritional control of emotional, physical and intellectual cognition, to get you working on your EPIC performance. Although this is a complex subject, there's also no reason not to keep it simple, and that's what we shall do. The nutritional forces you discover in the next several chapters may surprise you.

Neural Nugget #2 – Fish Food

The Skinny On Important Fat

Omega-3s work in concert with another type of polyunsaturated fat, called omega-6s. They are both essential, meaning we can't make them from scratch and have to eat them. You hear a lot about omega-3s these days, but not much about omega-6s. Why is this?

Our body and brain function optimally when omega-3s and -6s are kept in balance. They have many opposing functions and compete with each other for biological processes. For example, omega-6s are needed to kick-start some immune responses, like inflammation. Omega-3s, on the other hand, work to inhibit inflammation and keep the immune system in check. They are both crucial because you need to mount an immune defense against germs, but you also need to be able to keep it under control so that your immune system doesn't destroy your own cells and tissues.

Throughout most of man's history, back to our hunter-gatherer days, we seemed to eat a diet fairly balanced in omega-3s and -6s. The optimal ratio for these nutrients is about 1 to 3, give or take, in slight favor of omega-6s. However, today's typical western diet is about 1:20, with way too many omega-6s compared to -3s. This is why omega-3s are getting all the press. We need more omega-3s in our diets and less omega-6s.

How did this happen? If you look back in time, you find that we ate a lot of fish and game. Fish is high in omega-3 and so is grass-fed beef and chicken. The fish get their omega-3s from the marine algae and cows and chickens get them from eating grass. Omega-6s, on the other hand, are high in many vegetable oils (especially corn oil) which are major components of all the processed foods we eat. Not only that, but beef and chicken raised mostly on corn meal, as is common today, have much higher levels of omega-6 in their meats than do their grass-fed counterparts.

So it's easy to see why today's western diet is out-of-whack when it comes to omega-3 and omega-6 ratios. We simply eat too many sources of omega-6s and not enough of omega-3s. This potentially leads to an over-active immune system and inflammation, a condition that likely underlies many of the chronic degenerative diseases we are plagued with today. For example, heart disease, some cancers, Alzheimer's disease and many others often have inflammation problems at their root.

Furthermore, when it comes to the brain omega-3s play another role. In fact, brain tissue has a higher concentration of omega-3s than most other tissues in the body (along with eye tissue and sperm). Omega-3s are very important components of the cell membrane that we talked about above. Brain cells connect and talk to each other, but they do so in a very 'fluid' way. They aren't hard wired, like electrical wiring, but are flexible, more like Jell-o. This flexibility is required in order to make new connections and learn things.

Omega-3s contribute to the brain's physical flexibility and the less omega-3s in the brain cell membranes the more rigid and stiff they become, decreasing their ability to communicate efficiently. Also, research shows us that diets low in omega-3s can alter the levels of specific signals in the brain (dopamine and serotonin) that are involved in regulating mood. In fact, studies show that omega-3s are lower in the blood of people who attempted suicide and omega-3s are now being studied as a potential antidepressant.

On a final note, it merits mention that there are three main types of omega-3s and they have different roles in the body. The shortest of the omega-3 fats comes mostly from plant sources, like walnuts and flaxseed. This type, called ALA, can be beneficial for some diabetic patients by helping to increase sensitivity to insulin.

Specific machinery in the body can lengthen ALA to form another omega-3, called EPA, which is further lengthened to form the omega-3, DHA. However, this process of lengthening the omega-3 chain does not work very well in humans, but you can get the long chain forms directly by eating fish. EPA has a big role in keeping the vascular system healthy and DHA is the one that plays a big role in the brain.

This is important because it's difficult to get all the brain-boosting affects of omega-3s strictly from grain and nut sources. Fish is really the best.

All in all omega-3s play a role in many brain functions; from regulating mood to increasing cognitive abilities. These reasons put foods rich in omega-3s near the top of the list for a brain healthy diet. See the appendix for a look at foods high in omega-3s and omega-6s.

CHAPTER 3

FOOD FOR MOOD

Nourish Your Emotional Intelligence

"Although there is a great deal of controversy among scientists about the effects of ingested food on the brain, no one denies that you can change your cognition and mood by what you eat."

- Arthur Winter (author, inventor and neurosurgeon)

When we talk about nutritional regulation of your emotional intelligence, we are largely talking about a few things: your ability to handle your own stress, stay out of a prolonged depressed state, and generally improve your sense of well being. Everyone has sad times and that is normal. But if you continually find yourself down and lethargic you should consider making some changes or getting some help. In this section, we'll discuss the roles that various nutrients have on the psychological and physical aspects of mood and response to stress.

Our idea that nutrition plays a role in mood regulation dates all the way back to Hippocrates in 400 B.C. with his statement, "Leave the drugs in the chemist's pot if you can heal the patient with food." This attitude was still prevalent in the western world in the earlier part of the 1900s. The *Peoples Home Library*, published by Ritter in 1910, was a common source of medical information in a time when medical advice was not just a mouse-click away. This book clearly cited "imperfect nutrition" as the number one cause for "acquired insanity". Even as recently as the 1940s, nutritional deficiency had an accepted role as a primary factor in psychiatric illness.

However, in the mid-1900s, the discovery of pharmaceuticals that could effectively treat mental illness quickly diverted research attention and funds to a more 'molecular' hypothesis of mental health. This direction was solidified by the clinical success of antidepressants that increased serotonin, dopamine and norepinephrine in brain circuits associated with mood. Today, there is little doubt that these neurotransmitters play a big role in aspects of mental health, and manipulating them with drugs can be effective in some patients. The question that remains though, relates to why these neurotransmitters need fixing so frequently in society today. This is where nutrition, as well as the other cornerstones of brain fitness, comes back into the picture.

Unfortunately, once we develop a treatment for a given illness, prevention often seems to go out the window. In fact, we have had a difficult time integrating treatment and prevention throughout most of our history. Even back in Greek mythology, the story says, Aesculapius (the Greek god of medicine) spent most of his time keeping his two daughters from fighting. One was Hygeia, the goddess of prevention and the other was Panacea, the goddess of cure. The pages in this chapter will discuss how certain foods and nutrients control the activity of brain chemicals that control mood, and how attention to nutrition has a role in prevention *and* treatment of mood disorders.

Food For Your Mood

Everyone has heard of comfort foods. This usually refers to foods that you crave when you need a little pickup, or that conjure up safe and happy feelings with which that food has been associated. For most people these sweet or fatty foods taste good and give them an instant sense of stress relief. We're not promoting that kind of eating in this section, but it does have its occasional benefit and we'll discuss that a little later on. We'll also get into the brain circuits that are responsible for those feelings of pleasure and give you a better way to use food to help manage your mood all the time, not just in those desperate situations. Paying attention to nutrition can help you regulate your everyday mood experience.

One trick is to stay out of deficiency for any major nutrient that can affect your mood. Your brain has a way to figure out what nutrients it hasn't been getting enough of, and will crave foods that provide a 'quick fix' for the ones it is low in. For example, if you're low on energy because of a drop in glucose (blood sugar crash) you may crave something very sweet, like cakes or cookies. We want to avoid those deficient states to keep those cravings to a minimum.

In addition to a physical deficiency of some nutrients, you may also experience psychological cravings for foods that you know, through experience, make you feel better. You have learned to associate pleasure, or the relief of sadness, with certain kinds of foods. Avoiding deficient states can help stave off these cravings as well, because you will be less likely to enter the emotionally susceptible state that leads to psychological craving in the first place. To be clear, we are not saying that nutrition is the sole factor that regulates how you feel or what you crave. Mood is a highly complex thing that we still don't completely understand. However, nutrition certainly plays a role and the more you pay attention to some simple concepts, the greater your odds for staying emotionally stable and the better you'll be at handling the day-to-day stressors that life throws at you.

Comfortably Numb

In western society, we use comfort foods frequently to attempt to elevate our mood. In the short term, there may be some beneficial effect of these foods from the perspective of reducing stress. However, in the long-term they can be problematic. Many folks in our society find themselves faced with a lot of stress all of the time. We don't typically have the same stressors that we used to (or that many people in undeveloped countries face). Most of us don't worry about basic survival needs, like food, water and shelter. However, we do tend to worry about a lot of other stuff related to jobs, our kids, paying the bills, or who will become the next American Idol.

Comfort foods temporarily dampen the stress response by turning down the hormones that are making you feel stressed. Food affects the way you feel, and that affects the hormones that surge though your blood and brain to control your mood even further. If comfort foods were an occasional self-treatment, they probably wouldn't be a big deal and may even be beneficial for stress control. This also makes sense from a historical perspective. If you've been chasing a wooly-mammoth around for a week before you could finally catch and eat it, think of how rewarding that meal must have been! However, our immediate access to comfort foods all the time encourage us to over use this method of dealing with stress and this eventually leads to weight gain and other health problems. The irony is that putting on extra weight actually contributes to your physiological stress and increases the stress hormones that you were trying to reduce with comfort foods in the first place.

The bottom line is that there is a big difference between having a couple of squares of dark chocolate after dinner (no one can eat just one) to give your brain a little dopamine surge and pick up your mood, versus binging on a half a box of Oreos every day at the office. You can really liken comfort foods to alcohol use. Moderation is OK, maybe even beneficial, but overuse is definitely problematic. There is a much better approach to using food to combat stress and depression that we'll talk about in this chapter. In the pages that follow, we'll get into some specific foods and nutrients that are known to help your brain regulate your emotions. In later chapters, we'll also discuss how physical and mental activity, as well as sleep play important roles in this aspect of your EPIC performance.

Power Your Will With Steady Blood Sugar

The first and most simple concept we want to discuss centers around using low glycemic foods to temper your cravings. We talked about the glycemic index in chapter 2. Essentially, you want to eat foods that burn slowly and don't spike your blood sugar. These are whole grains, fruits and vegetables (with plenty of fiber) lean protein and healthy fats. The glycemic index is important for your brain's control of your emotions because a steady supply of glucose to the brain helps you deal with stress and stave off unhealthy cravings that can get you into trouble.

If your brain finds itself low on its fuel source, glucose, it will immediately activate brain circuits that stimulate hunger, and specifically crave high sugar foods. In the days of our ancestors, these foods would have been fruits and grains. But today we have taught ourselves (consciously or not) that Twinkies and donuts are loaded with the energy our brain desires and have the added benefit of activating our pleasure centers at the same time. This leads to an association of a positive emotion with eating these foods and creates a cycle of poor nutrition. Obviously, this is not the ideal method to deliver sustained energy to the brain.

In fact, many studies show a very real elevation in mood following high sugar, simple carbohydrate meals. High carbohydrate breakfasts raise blood sugar quickly and provide an elevation in mood and energy within about 15-60 minutes. The problem is that about two hours after a high carbohydrate meal, blood sugar is on its way down again – and it's falling hard. This leads to much lower mid-morning energy than eating a better mix of proteins and carbohydrates in the morning. Recent studies have also shown that we are most susceptible to the blood sugar rise and crash with a high carbohydrate breakfast, than we are at lunch or dinner. Furthermore, it appears some folks are especially prone to exhibit severe irritation and aggressive behavior during a blood sugar crash. You'll be very familiar with these types of mood swings if you live with one (or more) of these people.

You can combat these sugar cravings in a couple of ways. First, reset your brain to crave fruits, grains and slow burning foods, by making the lifestyle adjustment to focus on low glycemic eating. Second, don't let yourself get too hungry in the first place. Studies show us that if you let your blood sugar drop too much you lose a lot of will power and start seeking the quick fix. This is why you should always eat before you go grocery shopping, you'll be amazed at your ability to resist impulse buying, and how much easier it is to avoid buying junk food. Nutritionists have been touting the benefits of frequent small meals for years. This is one reason. Eating small and often keeps your brain out of an energy crisis so you don't experience the urge to binge. Furthermore, when you find yourself faced with those morning office donuts, you have the mental energy to walk on by. These adjustments take time if they are not already part of your routine so you shouldn't expect to master this change just because you read this paragraph. However, small steps over time eventually become habits, and habits become lifestyles and that is the ultimate goal.

Now let's get into a couple of specific nutrients that have a mountain of data supporting their essential role in regulating your mood, helping you deal with stress, and keeping depression at bay.

Fish Food For Mood Dude

One of the best-studied classes of nutrients relevant to psychological stress is, again, the omega-3s. We discussed the basics of omega-3s in chapter 2. In this section, we get into some of the roles they play in stabilizing your mood.

There are many studies connecting dietary omega-3 intake to various aspects of mood. In general, societies that eat more fish, the primary source of the brain healthy omega-3s (EPA and DHA) have lower rates of depression. There are also seasonal variations in suicidal behavior that correlate with fish intake. In Scandinavian countries, during times of the year when fish intake is lower, there is an increase in violent suicides. In some studies, people that attempted suicide, have lower blood levels of omega-3s and in other studies people with less fish intake admitted to considering suicide more frequently. Now, this is not to say that if you don't eat fish you will find yourself perched on top of a bridge, but, combined with other life factors and genetic drivers, omega-3s do seem to play a strong role in regulating mood and depression in many people.

All of these human studies provide strong circumstantial evidence that omega-3 intake affects mood. But the human data are still circumstantial, meaning we can't conclude from them that low omega-3 intake *causes* depressed moods. That's where rodent studies become beneficial because they provide a greater degree of flexibility to see if low levels of dietary omega-3s can actually contribute to mood disturbances. Neuroscience researchers use rats and mice because they have many of the same basic brain circuits as humans. They lack the large cortex that we have, the part of the brain responsible for higher levels of thinking, reasoning and self-awareness. However, they do have many of the same circuits that control learning and memory, and the underlying circuitry that controls emotion, mood regulation, and even addictive behaviors.

In rats, researchers can look at dopamine and serotonin in relation to their level of depression or anxiety. Serotonin and dopamine are two important neurotransmitters that play a particularly large role in depression and anxiety in rats and humans. More dopamine in certain areas of the brain usually means greater pleasure sensation and serotonin is linked to many things, including stress control. In fact, most of the antidepressants on the market today target increasing dopamine and/or serotonin activity in the brain (along with another neurotransmitter called norepinephrine). Researchers can evaluate dopamine and serotonin levels, and depression and anxiety behavior in rats, after altering the omega-3 content of their diet.

We know, what you're thinking. How can you tell if a rat is depressed or anxious? It's not like you can lay them down on a couch and interview them. But rats do have behaviors that indicate whether or not they are anxious or experiencing something similar to depression. For anxiety, researchers look at the desire of rats to explore new environments. Less exploratory behavior is associated with higher anxiety. Rats are social and exploratory creatures. If they are unwilling to check out new places, especially if it contains a tasty food or a buddy, then they appear to have an anxiety problem.

For 'depression-like' behavior, researchers can look at a rat's interest in pleasurable things, like sugar water. 'Anhedonia' is a lack of interest in doing tasks to gain a pleasurable reward. In humans, anhedonia is prevalent in many depressed subjects. Depressed people are often not that interested in seeking pleasure. Rats typically love sugar water. If a rat shows anhedonia, it is unwilling to perform a simple learned task to get some of the sweet stuff, so this is one depressive-like behavior to look for. Researchers can also look at a rat's effort to get out of a tank of water because they really don't like to swim. This is typically done during a very short 5-minute test. A normal rat will try to climb the walls, looking for a way out, whereas a 'depressed' rat will give up easily and just float.

If you deplete a rat's diet of omega-3s you see a decrease in serotonin and dopamine activity in parts of the brain that control mood. If you supplement omega-3s or put them back into their diet, you increase serotonin and dopamine activity in those mood-controlling brain areas. Furthermore, if you test these rats for depression-like or anxiety behaviors you see that rats deficient in dietary omega-3s are more depressed and more anxious than those who were given omega-3s in their diet. These studies provide a nice link between eating omega-3s and the brain chemistry that controls mood. So, even though the human data are circumstantial, the rodent data supports the idea that there are direct links between omega-3 intake, brain chemistry, and mood.

Studies suggest that a good dose of omega-3s for people is about an average of 1 gram (EPA + DHA) per day. This is equivalent to about three servings (3-4 ounces per serving) every week of a high omega-3 fish, like sardines or mackerel; or a daily serving of a lower omega-3 fish, like pink salmon or tuna (see table for omega-3 content in fish). Of course, these days we also have to consider how much mercury we get from eating too much fish. Still, you can get a good dose of omega-3s without exceeding the recommended limits of mercury consumption. Unfortunately, since we have contaminated a major important food source, we will have to live with this trade-off until we come up with a plan to clean it up.

Source	Grams omega-3s per 100 gram serving
Sardines	3.3g
Mackerel	2.5g
Atlantic Herring	1.6g
Chinook Salmon	1.4g
Anchovies	1.4g
Atlantic Salmon	1.2g
Bluefish	1.2g
Pink Salmon	1.0g
Florida Pompano	0.6g
Tuna	0.5g
Brook Trout	0.4g
Shrimp	0.3g
Catfish	0.3g
Northern Lobster	0.2g
Haddock	0.2g
Flounder	0.2g

Modified from *Am J Clin Nutr* (suppl 4):1020-1031, 1997.

One good alternative is to take a high quality fish-oil supplement that totals about 1 gram of omega-3s per day. Just ensure that you get a supplement that has had the contaminants purified away. You can look on the label for some statement about purification. Many will say 'molecular distillation', which is an effective procedure to remove the toxic contaminants away from the beneficial omega-3s. All in all, the data are very strong that omega-3s can affect your mood and you should strive to get them into your diet.

B Complex, But Keep It Simple

Another class of nutrients strongly linked to mood and depression are the B vitamins. There are many causes of depression and we are not implying that all depressed patients are deficient in the B vitamins or that B vitamins are useful in treating all cases of depression. However, there are depressed patients who have B vitamin deficiency, and this seems to be a factor in their illness. This is especially true for folks who battle their first bout of depression in their older years, called late-life depression. Furthermore, a subset of depressed patients that don't respond well to antidepressant medication are often helped with B vitamin supplementation.

Folate and vitamin B12

Folic acid (also called folate or vitamin B9) and vitamin B12 have been the subject of the largest number of studies related to nutrition and mood regulation. Piles of data link low levels of B12 and folate in the blood to depression. Conversely, increasing folate and B12 seems to help treat depression. Without getting into all of the complex neurochemistry, folate and B12 are involved in the synthesis of the neurotransmitters dopamine, serotonin and norepinephrine. If you remember these from a previous section, you realize that they play a major role in the brain circuits that regulate mood and that many antidepressants raise the level of these neurotransmitters. Low dietary folate and B12 seem to contribute to lowering the levels of these important mood-regulating molecules. Conversely, adequate dietary intake of the B vitamins seems to normalize their levels in the brain. In fact, you may know someone who gets B12 injections for energy.

Also, inadequate dietary intake of B12 and folate leads to elevated levels of homocysteine in the blood. This is a nasty little molecule associated with increased risk of cardiovascular disease and stroke. In fact, many studies indicate that this is one way that low B vitamins contribute to depression. Elevated homocysteine can increase oxidative stress because it oxidizes easily and can lead to the formation of free radicals. We discussed how oxidative stress and free radicals damage brain cells and blood vessels in chapter 2, so you can see how this could cause problems. Additionally, by causing oxidative stress and increasing vascular disease, homocysteine can decrease the efficiency of blood supply to the brain and cause all kinds of issues, from depression to dementia.

Adequate levels of folate and other B-complex vitamins also provide a good example of the interaction between genetics and diet. A common gene variant alters a key enzyme that processes folate, called MTHFR (methyltetrahydrofolate reductase, however some people see an expletive with that acronym). This genetic difference can make the whole folate processing system more or less efficient, and affect the amount of folate that you need to get into your diet. This is one of probably hundreds or thousands of genetic variations that interact with nutrition to regulate your health; and is a major reason why there is no diet optimal for everyone. In rare cases, people can have a genetic abnormality that interferes completely with the ability to process folate. These people will have elevated levels of homocysteine, even if they get plenty of folate in their diet, and will develop a host of severe mental and physical problems. These cases move out of preventative nutrition and into the need for medical intervention.

To summarize, folate and vitamin B12 are directly involved in the synthesis of mood-regulating neurotransmitters, and are indirectly involved in brain health by keeping the vascular-damaging homocysteine levels low. So where can you get a good dose of this important class of vitamins? Folate is high in many green vegetables, like spinach and asparagus, and also lentils and garbanzo beans. Due to the major importance of this nutrient, many food manufacturers also fortify cereals and breads with folate. Vitamin B12 is high in some shellfish, like mussels and clams. Of course, a high quality multi-vitamin can help you get adequate doses of each of these nutrients as well.

Thiamin (vitamin B1)

The ancient Chinese characterized beriberi as early as 2600 B.C., which results from thiamin deficiency. This affects cardiovascular, muscular, nervous and gastrointestinal systems. The focus of this chapter is not to discuss severe deficiency requiring immediate medical attention, but to focus on sub-optimal levels of nutrition that can surface as mood and emotional disturbances. Many studies suggest that insufficient thiamine intake can have this effect. Inadequate thiamine intake associates with depressed mood, fatigue, introversion, lack of self-confidence, irritability, and general lack of well-being. Greater deficiency also seems to induce major depression, hypochondria, hysteria and anorexia.

Again, different people will be susceptible to different levels of inadequate thiamine intake before noticing one or more of the above symptoms. The best thing to do to ensure the best chance of maintaining a stable mood is to get enough of this and all the other nutrients we discuss. Some good sources of thiamin are wheat germ cereal and other fortified breakfast cereals, pecans, walnuts, lentils, peas and long-grain brown rice. Thiamin is also readily available in supplement form and a standard component of any quality multi-vitamin.

<u>Vitamin B6</u>

With all of the studies focusing on the role of B-complex vitamins, B6 has also received some attention. B6 is involved in the synthesis of the neurotransmitters, serotonin and norepinephrine, which you recognize by now as playing a big role in mood regulation. Several studies have looked at the role of using B6 to treat depression. However, the findings are not as strong as for the other B vitamins discussed above, with one exception. Studies that focused on pre-menopausal women consistently found a positive role for vitamin B6 in treating depression, while studies in men were much less convincing. These studies suggest that there may be some mood-regulating benefit to increasing vitamin B6 intake in women with moderate to severe pre-menstrual syndrome or depression induced by birth control pills. Some good sources of B6 include fortified cereals, bananas, hazelnuts, spinach, vegetable juice, chicken, turkey, or salmon. Again, vitamin B6 is available in supplement form and found in adequate doses in quality multi-vitamins.

Other Vitamins

Other vitamins also show some correlation with depression but the data are a little sparse. One study showed that people with depression had lower levels of vitamin E in their blood, but no studies have attempted to treat depression with vitamin E supplementation as of yet. A few studies have also looked at the use of multi-vitamins in preventing or treating depression. The problem with these studies is that the term 'multi-vitamin' can mean so many things and the majority of commercially available products are not of high quality, as discussed in chapter 2. This makes it difficult since many of the studies are really comparing apples to oranges, so to speak.

However, there was an interesting study published in 2007 in *Clinical Nutrition* looking at the effect of supplementing a few hundred older adults during an extended hospital stay. All of the adults in the study remained on regular hospital food, but half received a placebo supplement and the other half received a multi-vitamin and multi-mineral complex. This allowed researchers tight control over what all the subjects were eating and supplementing. After six weeks, the folks taking the vitamin scored significantly better on measures of depression. A particularly disturbing finding of this study was that the blood levels of vitamin B12 and folate for the people on the hospital diet alone, actually went down over the course of the six week intervention. This doesn't say much for the nutritional value of this particular hospital's food.

Minerals

Several minerals make the list of things affecting the way you feel. Given that psychiatrists have been using the mineral, lithium, to treat depression for decades, this shouldn't really come as a big surprise. Topping the list is calcium. This is an incredibly important mineral that we need to get daily in relatively large amounts. Much of our physiology, including our cardiovascular, muscular, skeletal, and nervous systems rely heavily on calcium to function at all. Calcium is so important to our survival that we have dedicated an entire food group to it, incorrectly labeled the 'dairy group'. You can survive just fine without dairy, but not without some source of calcium. Yes, dairy is a good source of calcium but it is not the only source and our government should not promote it as such. Okay, enough of that particular soapbox.

Inadequate levels of calcium have been associated with depression and other mood disturbances in many studies. Again, some of the strongest data applies to helping pre-menopausal women regulate mood during premenstrual syndrome. Other studies also relate calcium imbalance to depression in a wide variety of men and women. However, it's unlikely that dietary insufficiency accounts for all calcium imbalance. Many factors, including genetic and other dietary components affect calcium metabolism. One nutrient that may be problematic in today's society is the effect of insufficient vitamin D intake on calcium absorption through the gut and calcium transport throughout the body. If you don't get enough vitamin D in your diet, you can't use the calcium that you eat as efficiently. This is an important consideration because emerging data indicate that vitamin D deficiency is rather widespread, making this a current hot topic for public health policy.

Other Minerals

Selenium, zinc, chromium and magnesium deficiencies have all been associated with mood disorder, including depression and aggressive behavior. These minerals also have been successful in some clinical trials in combination with antidepressant or anti-psychotic medication. From a global perspective, iron deficiency is a prevalent nutritional concern, especially during early childhood because of its strong role in brain development. Hemoglobin relies on iron to transport oxygen through the bloodstream to all brain and body tissues. A lack of iron can starve tissues of oxygen delivery required for the energy production that we discussed in the opening chapter of this section.

Moving On

In the next chapter, we'll explore the role that nutrition plays in helping your brain control your body. You'll find out which concepts and approaches give your brain the best odds of getting your body performing at optimal levels now, and keeping it going that way as you age.

CHAPTER 4

MIND, BODY & FOOD
Nutrition For Mind-Body Control

"Leave your drugs in the chemist's pot if you can heal the patient with food."
- Hippocrates, circa 400 B.C. (father of medicine)

As we discussed in the opening chapter of this book, the physical intelligence (PQ) of your brain is the ability of your brain to appropriately respond to and instruct the rest of your body organs and systems. This chapter discusses the role of nutrition in maintaining, regulating and optimizing your PQ. Your brain sends out chemical and electrical signals to instruct the other organs in your body. It is also 'listening' to the chemical signal output from those organs. This means that in order for your brain to exert *appropriate* control over your heart, lungs, liver, spleen, fat stores, immune system, etc., they need to output the right signals themselves. Nutritional factors play a large role in this interaction.

Your brain and your body are communicating in a couple of major ways. First, there are direct connections between the neurons in your brain and the nerves in your organs. This 'innervation' runs between your brain and the organs and tissues of your body, through your spinal column. Second, *hormones* travel through your blood stream to send messages between your brain and body. Both of these methods are two-way communication lines. Your brain sends messages via nerves and hormones to your body tissues, and they send messages back to the brain by the same means.

The accuracy with which these communications take place, is what we refer to as your physical intelligence. Think of this dialogue between your brain and body organs like conversations you have with other people. You may have had occasions when you have said something to a friend that they completely misunderstood. You 'emitted' one message but they 'received' something different. This may have happened the other way around as well. Your friend said something that you took wrong. Sometimes this happens by choosing the wrong words. Sometimes it happens when one person changes the topic or context while the other is still thinking of something else. Sometimes you receive mixed messages that seem to mean two contradicting things. Whatever the case the intended message is misconstrued and misunderstood.

These communication errors can also happen in the dialogue between your brain and body. For example, your brain or body organs could release an inaccurate chemical messenger into the blood stream. This could convey a message that simply isn't true, like 'I'm hungry' when you just ate. Messages may also occur in the wrong context when nerves fire or hormones release into the blood stream unnecessarily. For example, sometimes a nerve carrying a pain signal fires for seemingly no reason and gives you a brief painful sensation. The brain may also receive mixed messages. Your intestines tell your brain they are full of food but your eyes are sending images of dessert, creating an internal battle to eat or not.

To Eat Or Not To Eat

One of today's most relevant behaviors controlled by your physical intelligence is your drive to eat. Appropriate control over your appetite obviously affects your body weight, and this has dramatic consequences for much of the rest of your brain and body health. All the major chronic health problems that plague large portions of our society today are in some way related to body weight. Being overweight increases the probability of heart disease, diabetes, high blood pressure, Alzheimer's dementia, and a host of other problems. Because of this, we will spend a big chunk of this chapter on how to use quality nutrition to boost your PQ and regulate your food cravings.

The brain circuits that control feeding are highly complex and we still have a lot to learn about them. Still, there is a lot that we do know, and we will discuss how the *fitness* of this particular brain circuit has a huge impact on your overall brain and body health. Our brain circuits are hard-wired to ensure we eat enough to store energy. This is because our physiology was optimized in a time when food was relatively scarce. We needed to eat when we could and store that energy for lean times. Today, we rarely face lean times. Most people always have food available so those messages to eat high-energy foods whenever possible don't fit in our current environmental context. We need to 'train' our brains to adapt to our new context where food energy is typically abundant, which we'll get into in this chapter.

There are actually a couple of different types of hunger. First, there is 'homeostatic' hunger, which is hunger driven by low energy stores and a need to stock up. Homeostasis is a complicated term that simply means that your body tries to maintain itself in the same condition; 'homeo' means 'same', and 'stasis' means 'state of balance'. Think of it like the thermostat in your house. When it gets too hot, the air conditioner kicks on. When it gets too cold, the heater kicks on. Your thermostat is maintaining temperature homeostasis in your house; it keeps your house within a temperature range that feels comfortable to you. Your brain is attempting to do the same thing for all of your body functions, including body temperature, water balance, energy stores, etc. So if your brain senses low energy stores from not eating enough food, it will create a drive to eat by making you feel hungry.

Second, there is hedonic hunger. This is hunger simply for reasons of pleasure or sadness avoidance. Your energy stores may tell your brain that you're fine, but your pleasure centers are working hard to get you to indulge. Imagine that you just finished Thanksgiving dinner, stuffed to the brim with mashed potatoes, turkey and your grandmother's green bean casserole with bacon, but then you see the apple pie and ice cream. Suddenly, you feel a small pang of hunger. Your brain has received visual messages about the availability of some high-energy, pleasurable food, which it relayed to your hunger and pleasure circuits, and created a desire to eat it. It told your body you were still a little hungry, when that wasn't really true.

Different parts of your brain control these opposing behavioral drivers to eat for energy balance or to eat for pleasure. A small part of your brain, called your hypothalamus, is largely responsible for homeostasis. It is constantly checking your body temperature to keep you at 98.6; your salt and water balance to control your thirst; your blood sugar and other energy signals to control your hunger; your sleep-wake periods to control your daily cycles; and a host of other 'house-keeping' functions. Other parts of your brain, which mostly use the familiar neurotransmitter, dopamine, control your drive for pleasure, whether it's food, sex or rock and roll.

Back in the day when food was scarce, these two systems cooperated much better. You find pleasure in eating sweet and fatty foods because they are high in energy. In times of scarcity, this is a good survival instinct – eat as much high-energy food as you can, you never know when the next meal will be available. But today, this particular pleasure seeking behavior is working against your hypothalamus and its effort to

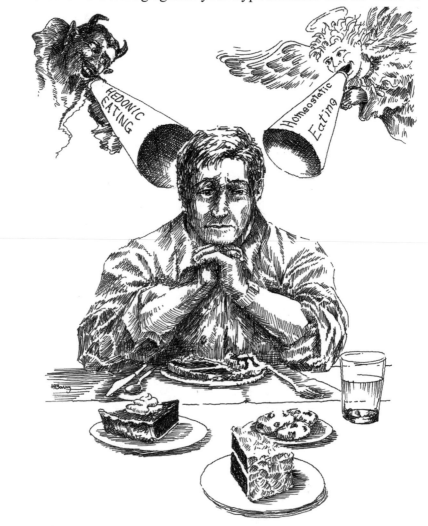

"Your hedonic pleasure circuits can be like the devil sitting on one shoulder, while your homeostatic eating circuits can act like an angel sitting on the other shoulder. A low glycemic diet can help prevent mixed messages from these two forces."

maintain energy balance. In today's environment, the pleasure-driven hedonic eating behavior is like the little devil whispering into your right ear, while the homeostatic-driven eating behavior is the little angel whispering into your left ear. For most of us, that little devil carries a much more attractive message.

Our goal is to get your pleasure centers to crave healthy behaviors, appropriate for today's environment. We want to get that little devil and that little angel telling us the same thing so we're not always battling unhealthy behaviors, at least most of the time. As we discussed in the last chapter, there is always a place for our favorite vices, as long as we keep them in moderation. Focusing on quality nutrition will help you get your health and brain fitness into an upward spiral instead of a downward one.

Nutritional Public Enemy #1

To begin the discussion on how to accomplish this we are going to return to the glycemic index. We'll assume that by now you have a handle on the basic concept of the glycemic index. High glycemic foods drive your blood sugar up fast. Low glycemic foods help maintain steady blood sugar levels. You can review chapters 1 and 2 for a more detailed discussion, if need be. Excess sugar, found in many high-glycemic foods, is public enemy number one in the battle to transition from unhealthy to healthy eating. Excess fat is a problem as well, but sugar cravings are the downfall of most people, from a behavioral standpoint. This is critical to the discussion of brain fitness because excess sugar is the main cause of Type II diabetes, and this disease associates with cognitive illness, like Alzheimer's disease, and emotional instability, like depression.

Physicians used to call Type II diabetes, 'adult onset' diabetes, because kids rarely got it. Today, more than half of the new diabetic cases in kids are Type II and the Center for Disease Control predicts that one out of three kids born today will become Type II diabetics at some point in their life. The biggest reason for this epidemic (and it does appear to be an epidemic) is poor diet along with lack of physical activity.

When you eat high glycemic foods and spike your blood sugar, your insulin rises to tell your body tissues to absorb glucose to bring your blood sugar down. If you do this too often, you may eventually become insulin resistant; meaning your body tissue will no longer respond efficiently to insulin, ignoring the message to take up sugar from your blood. This typically happens first in muscle cells, which need the most energy from sugar. At this stage of insulin resistance most of the sugar energy diverts to your fat cells, since they remain insulin responsive longer, and you start to gain belly fat.

As your insulin resistance gets worse, your blood sugar stays high and your pancreas needs to make more insulin to try to get it down. If this continues, your pancreas gets over-worked and eventually the cells making insulin can begin to burn out. Then you are well on the road to becoming diabetic. In many cases, this vicious cycle starts with too much sugar in your diet, making a focus on low glycemic eating imperative.

Here's the difficulty, however. As your blood sugar rises and insulin goes up, it also stimulates dopamine circuits in your brain to activate pleasure centers. This reinforces the message that the high-sugar food you just ate felt good, making you want to seek these foods in the future. In fact, recent studies in mice that lack the ability to taste sweet things show that sugary drinks activate dopamine-driven pleasure centers, even when they have no ability to taste the sugar. This is working below your level of consciousness. The rise in blood sugar is enough to trigger the pleasure centers, whether you are aware you ate something sweet or not.

This strategy to feel pleasure after eating high-energy foods ensures that we get enough energy, but in today's environment, it has turned into more of a curse than a blessing. The interaction between blood sugar, insulin and dopamine in the brain is a hot topic of research and not completely understood, but it is clear that sweet and high glycemic foods use dopamine brain circuits to create the feeling of pleasure.

So here's the rub. Your body is always trying to maintain homeostasis, or balance, as we have discussed. It does this by continuously turning up or down the activity of certain genes, which turn up or down the activity of certain brain circuits. This is to try to protect you from continually over-activating any given circuit. When you repeatedly activate pleasure centers with high glycemic foods, you tune down the degree to which they activate, so the pleasure sensations become less intense. So eventually you will need two teaspoons of sugar to get the same feeling of pleasure you used to get from one teaspoon of sugar (this is just an example, don't go around eating teaspoons of table sugar). You probably can't remember the first time you tasted chocolate ice cream, but your pleasure circuits likely lit up like a Christmas tree when you did. Now you may enjoy it (maybe even a lot), but the intensity has diminished.

If you eat high glycemic foods all the time, you will crave them to feel normal. The increases in blood sugar drive pleasure-center activity, but that tunes down over time. When you stop eating sugary foods, you just don't feel satisfied and you'll crave that sweet sensation. However, as you adjust your diet toward low glycemic foods, you can retrain your brain circuits to lose the cravings for sweet foods and move into a healthier lifestyle. When you talk to anyone who has seriously adopted a healthy lifestyle you'll find that it is not a battle for them. They enjoy healthy foods and behaviors and you can too.

For example, we have a friend (wink-wink), who used to love donuts, pies and cookies. He still enjoys a piece of pie (especially strawberry rhubarb) or a peanut butter cookie now and then, but he doesn't eat them very often. He's given up donuts completely – too many trans fats. The thing is, he doesn't miss them at all. He made a solid effort to remove sweet things out of his daily routine and he has literally lost his cravings for them. He used to put sugar in his coffee but now when he tastes coffee with sugar it seems overwhelmingly sweet. If he takes a sip of soda pop now, it tastes like syrup. It's no longer a battle to avoid these things, he simply doesn't want them. Undoubtedly, some people have a stronger sweet tooth than others do, but you will be amazed at how much you can reduce yours with a true focus on low-glycemic eating. You can find resources to help you with this task in the appendix of this book.

Before we leave this subject, we need to add a little clarification. Don't confuse low-glycemic eating with low-carb diets. Most low-carb diets are low glycemic because high glycemic carbs are what spike your blood sugar. However, as discussed previously, your brain relies exclusively on glucose (which comes from carbs) and you need to get enough to keep your brain happy. You can still get plenty of the carbs you need for your brain and maintain a low-glycemic diet by focusing on high-fiber, whole grain sources of carbohydrates. Let's not forget that fiber has some important benefits!

Nutrition Public Enemy #2

We have just discussed how continually eating high-sugar foods can eventually lead to a shutdown of the cells in your pancreas that make insulin. When these cells are operating normally they actually have sensors on them that monitor the sugar levels in your blood. Activating these sensors by increasing blood sugar is what causes your pancreatic cells to release insulin. Your brain also has a bunch of neurons that sense blood sugar. When a rise in blood sugar levels activate these neurons, they release different hormones that make you feel satiated in an attempt to get you to stop eating. However, a *high fat* diet for a prolonged period of time can get these neurons to shut down. When this happens, your brain loses a big part of its control over regulating your blood sugar levels. This (as well as many other reasons) makes excess dietary fat public enemy #2.

Too much fat in your diet obviously shows up around your gut, but it also affects your brain's control of the rest of your physiology. We discussed, in the introductory chapter to this section, the right and wrong kind of fat. To remind you, your brain is about 65% fat and you need good poly- and mono-unsaturated fats in your diet. But most people are loading up on saturated fat instead, which can go beyond negatively impacting your belly to wreak havoc on your brain's physical intelligence as well.

In fact, even a single high fat meal can have an effect on the way your nervous system responds to stress. Typically, a mild stress (like seeing a snake in the middle of the path you're walking on; or barely avoiding an accident on the freeway), will cause your brain to raise your blood pressure a little. A single high fat meal will increase the amount that your blood pressure rises, in response to mild stress. This is no big deal if it happens once in a blue moon, but continual high fat eating and continual over-reactivity to stress can eventually turn into a serious problem where your brain can no longer adequately control your blood pressure.

Growing Bellies And Shrinking Brains

It's no surprise that high sugar and high fat diets lead to more belly fat. The discussion above details the role that your brain and your PQ play in this. But there's more to the story that you should know. The more we learn about the role of obesity in chronic illnesses, the more we realize how bad the belly fat really is. This particular type of fat releases hormones that mess-up a lot of other systems in your body and increase your risk of developing high blood pressure, high cholesterol, insulin resistance, and inflammation. Physicians call this cluster of risk factors, 'metabolic syndrome'. Once established, metabolic syndrome increases your chances of things that can actually take you down, like heart disease and diabetes; and evidence is mounting that metabolic syndrome increases your odds of depression and dementia.

A recent review of scientific literature made a strong case for the relationship between metabolic syndrome and depression. So much so, that some psychiatrists want to rename major depression, 'Metabolic Syndrome – Type II'. Other studies have linked metabolic syndrome to increased odds for Alzheimer's disease. A recent 30-year study found that people who are obese in their forties had twice the chance of developing Alzheimer's disease in their 70s. It's clear that poor health of your body (largely due to disregarding the four cornerstones we discuss throughout this book), alters a huge array of hormones that feedback to the physical intelligence of your brain.

Fight, Flight And Think

Next to your brain, your immune system is the most complicated and 'smartest' system in your body, and has a huge impact on your overall health. Obviously, you need a healthy immune system to fight infections and even diseases like cancer. At the same time, an over-active immune system can attack your own body tissues and cause health problems. So the concept of homeostasis is very important for your immune system to keep it on its toes and ready to fight disease, but able to turn itself down when the battle is over. The brain and the immune system are in a constant dialogue to make sure this happens and nutrition plays a key role.

One major way that the brain stimulates immune activity is through activation of the stress axis. Stress can mean a number of different things. From a physiological perspective, stress is simply a disturbance in your body systems. As already discussed, your hypothalamus has a big role in trying to maintain homeostasis, so when it senses stress of any kind it attempts to help your body do whatever is necessary to deal with the stress to bring things back to normal.

The stressors of yesteryear included lions, tigers and bears, oh my! They also included potential starvation or serious exposure to the elements. These were life threatening and required immediate action to survive. If you were face to face with a tiger, your brain would activate your stress system and drive energy to all the muscles needed to get out of there. Your brain would also put your immune system on notice in case you were slashed and needed some emergency tissue repair. Then, after the situation had passed, your brain would tell your body to chill out and get back to normal.

Today's stressors are typically due to work, relationships or financial obligations. They don't carry immediate consequences of an early demise, but they can be just as deadly if you don't deal with them. One of the worst kinds of stress is the feeling that you are not in control of your own life. This can cause long-term, chronic activation of your stress system. In turn, chronic stress can keep your immune system working at higher than normal levels and cause damage to brain circuits and body tissues. Due to this interaction between psychological stress, immune function and long-term brain fitness, all of the nutritional issues we discussed in chapter 3, regarding mental health (your EQ), apply here. Anything you can do to keep your mood stable and your stress under control is good for your PQ as well as your EQ.

Stress today can also occur from an infection or an injury, in which case your brain sends out instructions to raise body temperature and activate your immune army. Having excess abdominal fat is also a physiological stressor, as discussed above. Belly fat sends out signals that cause increased immune activation and, over time, can be damaging to other tissues. This is another reason why obesity correlates with so many other chronic diseases. Nutritional approaches, as we have already learned, can go a long way in dealing with this type of stress.

A specific nutrient that requires revisiting in this context are the omega-3s and omega-6s. We mentioned in the *Neural Nugget #2, Fish Food*, following chapter 2, that omega-3s and -6s can have opposing effects on the immune system. Omega-3s tend to dampen immune activation while omega-6s tend to increase it. We also mentioned that we eat a much greater ratio of omega-6s to -3s than we used to. So what this translates to is a diet that is poised to chronically activate the immune system. The body uses omega-6s to make immune system hormones, called cytokines, which crank up immune activity and can damage other tissues. Whereas, omega-3s actually decrease some cytokine production and help keep the immune system in check.

This doesn't mean that cytokines are bad. They are necessary for fighting infections, cancers and other diseases.

Think of using weed-killers to control the unwanted weeds in your garden. They can work well to keep your flowerbeds looking nice. However, if you cranked out the weed-killer indiscriminately, you would kill all the flowers as well. Similarly, cytokines have an important job in our bodies, but over production of them (which can be caused by a high omega-6 diet) can cause unwanted damage.

In fact, one current theory of schizophrenia involves an over-active immune system. During development and through adulthood, the brain uses the immune system to keep unnecessary brain circuits trimmed. Your brain is always making new connections and testing them for usefulness. If they turn out to be of no use, or even causing problems, your brain dismantles them. Cytokines and the immune system play a role in this process. There is mounting evidence that a factor contributing to schizophrenia is an over-active immune system at crucial points in development. Researchers speculate that this may underlie some of the 'wiring' problems that schizophrenics suffer from.

Another issue related to the interplay between nutrition, immunity and brain health are sub-clinical food allergies. Many people go years or even decades with a minor food allergy that they aren't really aware of but that has chronic affects on their mood and physical health. Some researchers have even put forward the role of sub-clinical food allergies in autism, bipolar disorder and schizophrenia. There is much work yet to be done in this area but the notion is worthy of research attention, given what we know about immune system affects on brain function.

The most common are allergies to dairy, wheat, nuts or shellfish, but any food can carry a potential allergy. Some folks have obvious allergies that they are well aware of and avoid foods that cause those allergies at all costs. Yet many people have allergies that don't cause life threatening reactions but can affect them more subtly. If you suspect you just don't feel that well after eating certain foods you should try removing specific foods from your diet for a couple of weeks and see if it makes a difference. An allergy specialist can help you out.

Moving On

The next chapter gets into the meat of what most people associate with brain fitness, cognitive and intellectual function. Do you know which nutrients help you think more clearly? You're about to find out.

CHAPTER 5

FOOD FOR THOUGHT
Nutrition For Cognitive Function

"He who does not mind his belly will hardly mind anything else".

-   Samuel Johnson, circa 1750 (poet and writer)

This chapter deals with the affect that your diet can have on your cognitive abilities, like learning and memory, problem solving and general focused thinking. To be clear, we're not talking about major leaps in IQ test scores. In fact, IQ is a problematic and potentially dangerous thing to use to measure and evaluate people. Steven Jay Gould has a great book, called *The Mismeasure of Man*, which deals with the misuse of IQ tests and misevaluation of intellectual abilities throughout man's history. If you are interested in that topic, you should consider picking yourself up a copy.

Instead, we will discuss nutritional approaches to help you perform at your best, cognitively speaking. You have most certainly had days when you have woken up with a 'brain fog'. You find yourself slow to process conversations with people, easily distracted, unable to focus, and generally in a blah state. Other days, you feel on your game. You are quick witted, focused, creative and highly productive. As Brian Tracy says, "Some days you wake up and say, 'Good morning God!', while on other it's 'Good God, it's morning'". Sometimes, as you age you may find yourself spending more days in the fog as opposed to enjoying that clear-view you have on game days. Nutritional factors are one thing that can play a role in this balance to keep your brain at its cognitive best on a regular basis.

Data on the role of nutrition in cognitive function falls into two main categories. First, studies address the role of nutrition in optimizing cognitive performance in healthy youth and adults of all ages. Second, research evaluates specific nutrients in preventing or treating Alzheimer's disease and other types of dementia. As with anything else, an ounce of prevention is worth a pound of cure. Using lifestyle choices, including quality nutrition, to maintain a healthy brain and prevent dementia are much easier than attempting to reverse cognitive decline once it is well underway. Still, there have been some clinical successes using nutritional therapies to treat dementia, but we are far from a cure for Alzheimer's disease.

Derailing Dementia

Oxidative Stress And Dementia

A large amount of scientific data regarding nutrition and cognitive function focuses on the role of oxidative stress in age-related cognitive decline. Oxidation promotes, and anti-oxidants seem to prevent, cognitive decline as we age. Based on our discussion in previous chapters, this shouldn't really come as any surprise. Oxidative stress can damage tissues and when brain tissues are damaged, you can't think as clearly. Anything we can do to help prevent that damage should be beneficial to the brain. It is especially important for neurons to keep oxidative stress under control because these cells live much longer than other cell types, so are more susceptible to accumulating damage over a long period of time. Studies show that several nutrients with antioxidant properties seem to help prevent cognitive decline during aging.

<u>Spicing It Up</u>

One nutrient that has received scientific attention for its role in the ability to prevent cognitive decline and potentially enhance memory is curcumin. If you're a fan of Indian foods, you're probably eating this already since it's found in the curry spice, turmeric. In fact, turmeric has been a stable part of Indian herbal medicines for centuries. Interestingly, rates of Alzheimer's disease in India are reportedly much lower than in the United States. A related study showed that elderly Singaporeans (Singapore has a large Indian population) who ate curry on a regular basis performed better on cognitive tests than those who ate little curry. These are observational data, meaning we can't yet say the curcumin is responsible for these improvements in cognitive function and clinical trials are currently underway to test that. However, scientists have shown curcumin's ability to slow the progression of Alzheimer's disease in mouse models and reduce the associated decline in learning and memory tasks, which is encouraging data that speaks to curcumin's cognitive value.

Curcumin seems to apply to other aspects of cognitive fitness as well. Studies show that dietary supplementation with curcumin can protect against traumatic brain injury. It seems to have this effect by boosting the brain's ability to make one of its best 'fertilizers', called BDNF. This brings up an interesting concept that we like to call 'prehab'. Many of the lifestyle approaches we discuss throughout this book go beyond improving your performance today. They can also help prevent or reduce brain damage following an injury. This prehab approach makes any needed rehab following injury go a lot smoother. You'll learn more about BDNF and the prehab concept in the next section on physical activity.

Improving What You've Got While You've Still Got It.

As discussed in the introductory chapter to this section, nutrients can have a direct impact on the thoughts you think by controlling the levels of neurochemicals responsible for those thoughts. This applies to brain circuits that control cognitive abilities, as well as the emotional circuitry discussed in the last chapter.

<u>Fill Your Tank Early</u>

Let's start by revisiting some important advice you got from your grandmother – 'eat a good breakfast.' Study after study shows that kids who eat breakfast do better in school, period. This applies to adults in the workplace as well. Your brain relies exclusively on the sugar, glucose, as an energy source and you must feed your brain in the morning to optimize your power of focus. Your brain can only store enough glucose for about 10 to 15 minutes of operation. To ensure that your brain doesn't run out of energy it is continually getting a fresh supply from your blood. Your brain will always get first dibs on glucose so you don't have to worry about a total shut-down (except in times of extreme starvation). However, studies show that increasing the glucose availability to your brain by maintaining steady blood sugar levels can improve performance on memory tasks. One reason this occurs is that increased glucose availability can boost acetylcholine levels, which is a brain chemical important for learning and memory. When you're just sitting around doing nothing, increased glucose doesn't have much of an effect on acetylcholine. But when you're actively employing your noggin' at school or work, or letting Alec Trebek make you feel stupid watching *Jeopardy*, acetylcholine gets used up. Having a good supply of glucose on board can help keep the brain supplies high so you can continue to learn and remember.

Now, throwing down some donuts before you run out the door or send your kids off to school armed with Pop Tarts, won't do the job. Going back to the concept of eating low glycemic foods, you want to supply your brain with a steady supply of slow-release glucose, which you'll get from whole grain foods combined with a little protein. Although Pop Tarts and waffles may be easy and immediately satisfying, you're almost certain to experience an energy crash within a couple hours. If you want to give your kids an advantage at school or give yourself an advantage in the workplace, take the time to get a good low glycemic breakfast. In fact, a recent study showed that kids who ate a low-glycemic breakfast, compared to a high glycemic breakfast with equal energy load (calories) had increased focus, better memory and lower frustration levels 2-3 hours after eating. A similar study showed that lower glycemic foods improved memory performance in the elderly. While this type of study has not been conducted for adults in the workplace, it's almost certain that the same principles apply.

Fish Food For Thought

Beyond the short-term, hour-to-hour controls, several key nutrients have shown benefit in studies of cognitive performance. First off, the omega-3s return to the picture again. There are many studies showing the relationship between increased quantity of omega-3s in the diet and improved cognitive performance. This seems to apply to all ages since studies range from looking at infants and children to late-life adults.

Several researchers have evaluated the amount of omega-3s eaten by pregnant women and intellectual measures of their kids later down the road. A large study of 11,875 pregnant women found that those who ate more seafood, which is high in omega-3s, during pregnancy had kids who scored better on tests of verbal communication, social behavior and fine motor skills. In another specific study, women who ate cereal bars supplemented with the omega-3, DHA, had children who performed better on infant problem solving tests at nine months of age. Another study tested kids at four years of age after their mother's took omega-3 supplements during pregnancy and found the children had increased performance on IQ tests, relative to those who's mother's did not supplement with omega-3s.

Brain tissue is highly concentrated in omega-3 fats and they are required for normal development and maintenance of the central nervous system. Since the brain undergoes a rapid growth spurt in the third trimester of pregnancy, it makes sense that getting a good supply of omega-3s into the maternal diet can have beneficial effects for the children's cognitive performance.

The importance of omega-3s doesn't cease at the end of pregnancy. These fats are highly concentrated in breast milk and infants who are breast fed generally perform better on cognitive tests than those fed formula. As a comfort to those who chose not to breast feed, supplementation of omega-3s in formula, as is common today, can improve some early childhood visual and cognitive performance to equal breast fed children. However, it is generally agreed that breast-feeding is optimal for childhood development. Nature has already designed the perfect formula and it's unlikely that we'll top it.

Moving past childhood, omega-3s continue to play a role in cognitive performance throughout life. Older adults, who eat more fish, also show improved cognitive performance in many areas. A study of Norwegians in their seventies showed that the more fish these adults had in their diet, the better their performance on tests of memory, visual processing, attention, spatial orientation, and psychomotor speed. Interestingly, in this study, the less processed fish, the better. Those who ate mostly lean or fatty fish performed better than those who ate more processed fish or fish sandwiches.

Many studies have also shown that omega-3 supplementation can help improve focus and cognitive performance in kids and adults with Attention Deficit and Hyperactivity Disorders (ADHD). We don't really understand the relationship between omega-3s and this disorder. It's not that people with ADHD simply don't get enough omega-3s in their diet. They seem to have lower blood levels of omega-3s than people without ADHD, even if they get the same amount in their diets. So there is something going on with the processing of these long-chain fats that is currently a hot topic of research. Still, there have been some clinical successes in using omega-3 supplementation to help improve attention and focus in kids with this disorder.

Teaching Old Dogs New Tricks With ALA And Carnitine

A few additional nutrients that have received a lot of attention in the cognitive research world are carnitine, and alpha-lipoic acid, often abbreviated ALA. However, don't get this confused with alpha-linolenic acid, which is a short-chain omega-3 that is also abbreviated ALA. You're just going to have to read the label a little closer if you want to tell the difference.

Carnitine and ALA aid the function of mitochondria by quenching free radicals and boosting efficiency of energy production. If you remember from the introductory chapter in this section, mitochondria are the energy power plants inside all your cells. Neurons do a lot, and therefore require a lot of energy. To meet their energy needs, they rely heavily on mitochondria that must be in good working order. Carnitine and lipoic acid help keep your mitochondria in tip-top shape.

Although the jury is still out on whether supplementing lipoic acid and carnitine can help reduce symptoms of existing cognitive decline, the data are reasonably strong that they are useful in improving cognitive function in older adults who don't currently have dementia. Again, it's much easier to improve health and prevent illness while you're still reasonably healthy, than it is to reverse dementia once it takes hold.

Studies show that supplementing N-acetyl carnitine and alpha-lipoic acid in old dogs helps them learn new tricks. Dogs are a good model to study dementia, partly because they are easy to work with when studying learning. When researchers gave old beagles carnitine and lipoic acid supplements for 2 months they had an easier time learning new tasks and made fewer errors than those dogs given placebo. In human studies, centenarians (people over 100 years old) benefited from carnitine supplementation as well. Researchers gave daily supplements of another form of carnitine, called levocarnitine, to a group of centenarians and compared them to another group of centenarians who received placebo supplements. Members of both groups were 100 to 106 years of age. After six months taking two grams per day, the centenarians on the carnitine supplements experienced reduced physical and mental fatigue. They did better on cognitive tests, were more active during the day and increased the distance they could walk before tiring. This is an impressive result for such a late-life treatment.

Carnitine and ALA are currently at the forefront of research looking for nutritional approaches to prevent and even treat cognitive decline and dementia. They are both readily available in supplement form and are part of some high quality multi-vitamin/mineral complexes. Carnitine is a natural compound found in all mammalian species and is high in meats like beef and pork. Food tables for lipoic acid are not yet complete; however, it is abundant in many plant and animal sources. Spinach and broccoli are good sources of lipoic acid, as are animal sources, especially liver, heart and kidney. Haggis anyone?

Folic Acid And B12

We discussed folic acid and vitamin B12 in the last chapter due to their roles in mood regulation. They return to the scene in this chapter, with roles in cognitive function, potentially for the same reason. We discussed how insufficient levels of these nutrients could increase the levels of homocysteine in your blood and brain tissues. Since homocysteine is easily oxidized and can be toxic to brain cells, it can also have detrimental effects on cognitive function. Folic acid and vitamin B12 help to keep homocysteine levels low and protect the brain from its rampage. This is especially true for the elderly due to increased odds for dietary insufficiency and decreased absorption of B vitamins from the gut. Another risk factor for the elderly is that they tend to be on several medications, many of which can interact to make folate and vitamin B12 deficiencies worse.

To be clear, severe folate and B12 deficiencies are rare due to the fortification of many foods with these nutrients. However, even being on the low end of normal for an extended period of time can increase risk for cognitive problems. Many studies report that lower blood folate levels associate with decreased performance on cognitive tests across young and old, men and women. But the data are not entirely clear and still a hot topic of research. Some studies show a negative effect of too much folate. The problem is that there is no standard dose of folate and some studies use whopping amounts that you would never get from your food and multi-vitamin use. A quality multi-vitamin will contain 400-800 micrograms of folate, an amount that has shown benefit for improving cognitive performance. Yet some studies dose up 10,000 – 20,000 milligrams per day in volunteers and this dose is not always beneficial. The optimal amount of folate and vitamin B12 also depends on age, genetics and lifestyle. Until researchers work all this out, you are better off focusing on eating folate rich foods, discussed in the last chapter; and taking a quality multi-vitamin product.

Vitamins A, C, E And About A Thousand Other Nutrients

Several vitamins have potential roles in protecting you from cognitive decline. Those with the most research, beyond what we've already discussed, are the vitamins A, C and E. The biggest reasons for their positive affects seem to be simply due to their strong antioxidant properties. These vitamins are key components in keeping oxidative stress to a minimum by continually neutralizing free radicals, as we discussed in chapter 2. It should be noted that there is not a lot of data that these vitamins can *reverse* damage to improve dementia, but there is substantial evidence that they can prevent damage, and lower the risk of getting dementia in the first place.

Vitamin A is a fat-soluble vitamin and does a good job acting as an antioxidant in brain cell membranes. This is one nutrient that is incredibly important for normal brain function, but that you don't want to overdo, as it can be toxic in high levels. Many quality nutritional supplements will contain beta-carotene, instead, because your body can convert this to vitamin A as needed, so there is less concern about toxicity.

A large clinical trial recently evaluated the role of beta-carotene supplements in cognitive function. In this study, volunteers who took beta-carotene for 20 years performed better on cognitive tests than those who did not take the supplement. Another group in this study took beta-carotene supplements for only 5 years and showed no cognitive benefit. This study highlights the difficulty in assessing the value of nutritional supplementation over a short time period. Many nutrients are likely to have long-term effects that are not apparent in short studies. As research continues, it is likely that we will discover many long-term nutritional benefits of which we are not currently aware. This reiterates the point that early adoption of lifestyle choices is a much better approach to life-long brain health and fitness than waiting until there is a problem and then trying to fix it.

Research has also revealed a strong cognitive role for Vitamin E in maintaining a healthy vascular system. Vitamin E also is fat-soluble, making it an effective antioxidant in blood-vessel cells membranes to minimize oxidative damage to the neurovascular system that is responsible for supplying oxygen and other nutrients to the brain. As we've discussed before, a healthy vascular system is a big factor in a healthy brain. Critics of nutritional supplementation, however, have latched on to some vitamin E research to point out potential dangers of over-supplementation. Vitamin E is one of the very few vitamins that have shown some negative effects in a small number of clinical trials. A couple of studies show a small increase in the chance of lung cancer in people that supplement high amounts of vitamin E. However, this is most profound in smokers, not non-smokers. Our take on this research is that you would do well to give up smoking to reduce your chance of lung cancer, not vitamin E.

Vitamin C is a water-soluble nutrient making it easier for your body to get rid of so you don't really have to worry about over-dosing vitamin C unless you are mega-dosing beyond any normal supplementation routine. Vitamin C is highly concentrated in the brain and involved in many reactions, including energy production. In fact, you're brain will hold onto as much vitamin C as it can if the rest of your body is getting enough, which suggests the importance this nutrient has for brain function. It is a strong antioxidant that helps to minimize oxidative damage in the watery environments inside the cell, which the fat-soluble vitamins A and E can't get to very well.

The best sources for all of the vitamins we have discussed are fruits and vegetables. Everyone knows they should get plenty of fruits and vegetables in their diet, and we have covered a few of the reasons why. Not only do these natural foods contain vitamins and minerals, they also contain many other brain boosting nutrients, many of which we are only beginning to appreciate. You may have heard of polyphenolics and flavonoids. These classes of nutrients represent hundreds of different antioxidant compounds that have proven beneficial for the brain in numerous studies. The old adage 'an apple a day, keeps the doctor away' is largely true due to vitamins, polyphenolics and flavonoids in the fruit. This adage applies to blueberries, strawberries, oranges, grapes, etc. It also applies to vegetables like broccoli, spinach, peas, brussel sprouts, etc. We understand that not everyone enjoys fruits and vegetables, which is too bad. If you are not a fan you should make a commitment to trying as many different fruits and vegetables as you possibly can in order to find some that you like. There are so many different varieties it's almost impossible to dislike them all. The more variety of these nearly perfect foods you can get into your diet the better your anti-oxidant protection systems will be.

The Good Things In Life Can Be Good For You Too

Not all our vices necessarily fit cleanly into the 'bad for you' category. There are some things that we enjoy which have shown some clinical benefit. The trick for most of these is to follow the rules of moderation. Life is about enjoyment and we want to wrap up this chapter by emphasizing the enjoyment factor. So here are some 'enjoyable' studies that gleaned some media attention, mostly because they conclude what we want to hear.

A group in Spain has studied the effects of drinking beer on damage to brain cells caused by aluminum. It turns out the beer consumption, equal to about one beer a day, can be partially protective against the toxic affects aluminum salts, which research attributes to some cases of Alzheimer's disease. Several studies show cognitive benefits of moderate wine intake, defined as one to two glasses per day. While researchers continue to attempt to nail down the 'key ingredient' in wine responsible for this benefit, it's likely due to a host of different compounds that work best together in a nice Bordeaux, not in a pill. Dark chocolate is another culinary pleasure that has received positive scientific data, likely due to the benefits of flavonoids and polyphenolics, which we have discussed. Caffeine is a 'nutrient' that gets a lot of press on both sides of the issue. It is definitely an acute stimulant and can improve cognitive performance in the short term. But there are also data suggesting that long-term caffeine consumption can be protective against dementia.

The bottom-line when using any of these 'vices' is to use them in moderation if you enjoy them. Nothing fits cleanly into the 'good' or 'bad' category. Everything is about balance. Part of the benefit of moderate use of your favorite vices is that fact that they can relieve a little stress and make you feel good. If you feel you are dependent on over-use of anything in particular, or your friends and family have confronted you with a problem, then you should evaluate that. However, if you

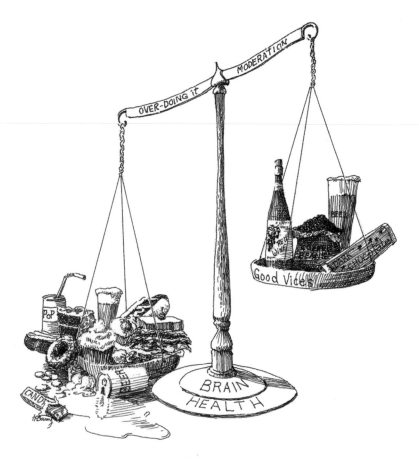

"Moderate use of your vices can be stress relieving and, sometimes, even beneficial. But overuse of the same things can quickly spiral out of control."

enjoy a glass of wine and a couple squares of dark chocolate in the evening – go for it.

Moving On

In the next section, we turn our attention to physical activity. It will help you boost your EPIC performance. When you combine the concepts of this chapter with those of the next, you'll more than double your benefits. But before we get there we will summarize the main concepts we have discussed throughout this section in the take-home message on the next page.

Summarizing The Nutritional Stew

As we said in the opening chapter to this section, there is no 'one-size-fits-all' diet for everyone. Your perfect diet depends on your genes, your activity level and the types of foods that you like and dislike. Still, when it comes to optimizing daily emotional, physical and cognitive performance, there are a few key points that are applicable to all. Here are some key concepts and action plans from this section.

Key Concepts:

- Nutrients are the raw building blocks for maintaining and building brain circuits.
- Oxidative stress, left unchecked, can damage brain tissues and a good diet with plenty of micronutrients and antioxidants can help protect you from that.
- Your brain is two-thirds fat and some fats (mono- and poly-unsaturated) are good and necessary for optimal brain function.
- Your diet affects the neurochemistry of your brain that controls mood and your response to stress.
- Your diet affects the way your brain talks to your body and vice-versa.
- Your diet affects higher brain functions that control learning, memory and intellectual function.

Key Action Points:

- Make as much of your diet low-glycemic as you possibly can. Make a special extra effort to get sugars out of your breakfast and replace them with whole grains and proteins. This will help you maintain your energy and your insulin sensitivity.

- Eat small and frequent meals everyday to feed your brain a steady supply of glucose. This will help keep your cravings to a minimum.

- Find a variety of different colored fruits and vegetables that you enjoy and work them into your diet – everyday. This will help minimize oxidative stress.

- Get your long-chain omega-3s by eating fish a few times a week. If you don't like fish, take a fish oil supplement. If you don't eat animal products at all, you can take an algae oil supplement to get your long-chain omega-3s. This will help your cardiovascular, neurovascular and neurochemistry to improve all aspects of brain fitness.

- Take a high quality multi-vitamin to fill in the holes in your diet. But remember they are supplements, not substitutes. This will help ensure you get a steady supply of needed micronutrients and keep you out of acute and chronic deficiencies.

- Don't give up everything that you enjoy, but keep your vices to moderate levels. This will help you deal with small levels of stress by giving yourself permission to indulge on occasion.

The Second Cornerstone

Physical Activity

CHAPTER 6

TAKING YOUR BRAIN FOR A WALK
Introduction To Physical Activity For Brain Fitness

"An active mind cannot exist in an inactive body"
- George S. Patton (US Army General)

Here's the overriding concept for how exercise impacts our brain's health: a body in motion tends to stay in motion. Since we've totally taken one of the main laws of physics out of context let us explain. This is really just another way to state the principle of 'use-it-or-lose-it' (UIOLI). I'm guessing that for most people the idea of UIOLI (pronounced you-e-oh-lee) is much more familiar in terms of our physical state (e.g. muscles) as opposed to our mental state. If you've ever been in a cast you understand completely. When the doctor cut that cast away you wondered what happened to your muscle. Inactivity for several weeks caused it to atrophy and it probably took you a lot of work and a long time to get those muscles back to their pre-injury capacity.

This principle clearly applies to your mental-self as well, and because your brain is the organ where perception occurs, UIOLI is exceptionally important for brain fitness. What we mean by this is that if your brain isn't functioning correctly, you may not even realize there is any loss in function because it's your brain that has to realize it. Sort of a 'tree falling in the forest' thing. If there's no one there to hear it, does it make a sound? If your brain isn't operating at full capacity, will it notice a small deficit? Sometimes a small loss of function may be obvious. This is especially true for changes in our ability to remember things as we age (which we'll get back to later). However, you may also experience subtle changes that you aren't aware of, which may eventually turn into major disabilities that everyone, including you, become aware of.

One of the most important things we'd like you to take away from this book is that there is a very tight link between your mind and body. For many people, the most obvious direction for this link may be the body-to-mind link. If you hit your thumb with a hammer, it hurts. This is your brain, your mind, perceiving signals from your body. A more difficult concept is how your mind influences your body, or the mind-to-body link. The way you perceive and think about things can affect your health. Stress causes the activation of your stress response, and one of the end points of this response is for your adrenal glands (small glands above your kidneys) to release the hormone cortisol. Cortisol is a very important part of your fright, flight or fight response and plays several other important roles in your biology. However, you are not meant to turn this hormone on at high levels for extended periods of time. Having tructions thels for long periods of time can actually do damage to your brain and body. This is one clear example of how your mind can affect your health.

What you cannot do is start to separate your mind's activity from your body. They play off and support each other. So really, your physical health is going to have an effect on your mental health and vice versa. This concept is most succinctly summed up with the line that We're sure many of you have heard, which is "the mind-body interaction." Interest in the mind-body interaction is starting to gain momentum in the research community, and scientific evidence that supports the idea is starting to accumulate. We talk about this extensively in chapter 12 in the discussion about mental activity and physical intelligence.

Physical activity or exercise (we'll talk about the distinction in a minute) influences how your brain functions. And these influences likely affect the function of both the mind-to-body and body-to-mind directions of the link. When you're thinking of exercise think about how road repairs are done. If you take a specific road to work that has a lot of potholes, you don't want them to just fix one side. If they do, your drive to work might be better, but your drive home will still be miserable. Luckily, exercise and physical activity seem to work on both sides of the road to benefit the two-way communication between your brain and body.

What Do We Need To Do?

We need to take a balanced approach to increasing our levels of physical activity. That is the short and bitter-sweet of it! You probably noticed in chapters 2 – 5 on nutritional approaches to brain fitness, there was a lot of ground to cover, a lot of options for tweaking your diet. But in terms of physical activity, it's very straight forward. The vast majority of us need more of it. What we'd like to do in this section is impress upon you the importance of increasing and maintaining physical activity levels for your brain's health, some strategies for incorporating physical activity into your daily routine, and some concepts for optimizing your efforts through appropriate timing.

As we mentioned above, there is a difference between physical activity and exercise. Many times you'll hear the terms 'physical activity' and 'exercise' used interchangeably, yet there is a subtle but important distinction between the two.

Exploring this difference will help you better assess where you are, and allow you to develop multiple strategies for achieving the goals you set for yourself.

Physical activity is an umbrella, or catch-all term, used to describe any action that requires muscle contraction in your body. Muscle contractions make your body move, or keep your balance and posture. This includes walking, chores, playing Wii sports, and in some cases even sitting (for example on an exercise ball; not so much if you're laid out in a Barcalounger). Exercise falls under the umbrella of physical activity and is a dedicated time for repetitive actions with the purpose of increasing performance or physical capacity. This is what most people think of when they hear the words physical activity and/or exercise and is probably what people tend to think of when they imagine what Olympians or professional athletes do on a day-to-day basis.

The best way to start as you begin to incorporate physical activity/exercise into your life is to do so slowly. Start with increasing your physical activity. This will help. For example, all the advice you've heard a thousand times before (but haven't followed yet): take the stairs instead of the elevator; park your car away from the store entrance; walk on short-distance errands instead of driving. It will be important, however, to eventually incorporate some *fitness-appropriate* exercise. Again, if you are new to this you should work with a professional and your physician to define a routine that's right for your level of condition.

Another idea we want you to accept is that you should strive for 'prehab' over 'rehab.' With prehab you build up your reserves, your health bank account that you can draw from on those rainy-days when you need a little extra cushion to protect your brain's health. If you are continually working on your physical health, when you do experience a little extra challenge, you will be much more capable of successfully dealing with it. The idea of reserve plays heavily into the concept of allostatic load that we discuss in *Neural Nugget #5, Shielding Yourself from Stress*. The reserve you build is a cushion, a back-up plan, or adaptations that we can make to help us work around problems that come up. We'll return to the concept of physical and cognitive reserves throughout this book.

The Way We Were

The title of this section stems from the title from of a fantastic album by the great jazz pianist, Dave Brubeck. The way we need to interact with our environment has changed drastically in the last 75 to 100 years, leading us from the way we were to the way we are.

If you look throughout the history of human kind, there have been very few times, if any, where the mass of society has lived with such a glut of resources while having to expend so little energy to reap these benefits. As we discussed in chapter 4 in the context of nutrition, our biology has developed to prepare for times of famine, and these adaptations have served us well, until recently. Here, we'll look at this same adaptation in the context of physical activity. In our current time, we have access to prepared foods that we can obtain with relatively little effort. Our day-to-day lives have also changed substantially in other ways over the last few decades to reduce our energy output. Since the implementation of the personal computer into most realms of school and work, and the advancements in entertainment technologies our daily activity levels have plummeted.

In the grand scheme of things, we have a biological inclination towards maintaining a positive energy balance. It makes sense when you think about it. Over the course of history we wouldn't have wanted to burn more calories than we ate, since we weren't all that sure when our next meal might be. We needed to conserve all the calories we could so we didn't starved to death. We've developed a lot of biological systems to ensure that we have access to enough calories (energy) when we need them. One way we do this is to turn the flame down on the burner so we conserve calories (energy), whenever possible. We are designed to conserve caloric energy, not burn it freely. Couple this drive to store energy with the massive recent reduction in the need to burn calories as part of our daily survival, and you have a recipe for weight gain.

The FAT Of The Land

We also have a much different landscape in terms of food. Home cooked meals are less common. Convenience and bargains have become the name of the game. However, we still have that drive for positive energy, which is to store more calories than we burn so we can pack some away for a rainy or drought ridden day. Since we're geared towards positive energy balance, and everyone knows that excess calories leads to increased body fat, we'd like to propose the acronym, FAT, standing for Fundamental Adaptation Towards positive energy balance. In this case, your FAT literally pushes you to accumulate fat so you will have a store of energy for tough times. Your degree of FAT is going to be influenced by your genetic makeup, but you do have a lot of control over your behavior and other factors that influence your drive to store energy. This is a case where you will have to make a conscious effort to help the autopilot parts of your brain know that there probably isn't a fast coming around the corner so you should probably pass up the third "double fudge, black forest, death-by-chocolate, whip cream-topped" milkshake of the evening.

In the past, the FAT portion of the equation probably wasn't that big of a deal since daily living required us to burn off a lot of those extra calories. Plowing the field, milking cows, feeding chickens, smelting iron, and saving damsels in distress, all required a fair amount of our energy. They definitely required more energy than Googling "how to smelt iron." But our environment has changed rapidly. The average person is far less physically active than even 50 years ago, and now we've run into a big problem. In fact, we routinely refer to the current level of obesity in industrialized nations as an epidemic.

This took time and likely occurred due to the combination of several factors (as we discuss in both the nutrition and sleep sections of this book) but today's relative lack of daily physical effort is certainly one of the big reasons. It has come to the point where we've actually become *deficient* in our levels of physical activity. The drastically lower levels of activity over prolonged periods of time has led many of us into our next acronym, PADS, which stands for <u>P</u>hysical <u>A</u>ctivity <u>D</u>eficiency <u>S</u>yndrome. This is an accumulation of choices that we make on how we're going to interact with our environment. Constantly searching for the easiest and least physically active way to do things. We drive hunting for a parking spot for ten minutes in order to save five minutes of walking. We have elevators, escalators and moving walkways to minimize our efforts. Not to mention, our choice to plop down in front of the TV after dinner instead of going for an evening walk. These poor choices lower our levels of physical activity in an environment that requires little physical activity from us to begin with. The good news is that PADS is something we have the ability to influence. Which is critical since, as we discussed above, FAT is hardwired into our biology.

If you consider the combination of the biological inclination and environmental choices we make, then we end up with FAT PADS, both figuratively and literally! Just to remind everyone that we're talking about a Fundamental Adaptation Towards positive energy balance, coupled with Physical Activity Deficiency Syndrome (FAT PADS), a double whammy! In years gone by, this was adaptive, since it prepared us for those inevitable periods of fasting or famine. We were able to store what we ate, due to our biology and decreasing our activity. But industrialized nations don't run into those periods of fast and famine all that often and with copious amounts of food and little necessity to be active, we have entered a state of epidemic obesity by our FAT PADS.

Can We Make The PADS Thinner?

The PADS idea is analogous to what happens with dietary deficiencies. There are numerous diseases caused by vitamin deficiencies that we can easily correct and practically eliminate by introducing the correct nutrient into the diet. Scurvy is an example of a vitamin deficiency, caused by insufficient vitamin-C, which is avoidable by introducing some citrus fruit into the diet. A couple of centuries ago this was a serious problem for people who embarked on long sea-voyages and many sailors suffered and died from this disease. In order to offset this problem the English Navy sent along barrels of limes, which is where the term "Limey" (slang used to refer to English sailors) came about. Rickets is a disease that results in abnormal bone formation and can result in severe bowing of the legs. Vitamin-D deficiency is the culprit here, which tends to occur most frequently in malnourished children. This deficiency can result in deformation of limbs and even fractures, but again, is avoidable with proper nutrition. Although this is much less common in developed countries like the United States, the number of affected children is much higher in developing nations.

Deficiency of the mineral, iodine, can lead to goiter. This is particularly problematic in inland areas where it is difficult or impossible to find seafood. Things like seaweed contain high levels of iodine, a trace element critical for proper function of our thyroid gland. To address this problem many countries have added Iodine to staple food products, like table salt (look at the bag in the store next time it will say *iodized table salt*), as a way to keep people from developing the disease. There are other causes of goiter that are more genetically driven, however most cases are due to Iodine-deficiency. It is estimated that in India 200 million people suffer from iodine-deficiency and 54 million have goiter.

Some of the most striking things about these diseases of deficiency are that they produce such debilitating symptoms, yet are so easy to address with proper nutrition or supplementation (e.g. vitamin and mineral supplements). We can substantially reduce the prevalence of the three deficiency related diseases mentioned above. When was the last time you saw someone with rickets or a goiter? It is very uncommon these days for those of us who live in industrialized nations. And we'd be willing to bet that 99.9% of people reading this book have NEVER met anyone with scurvy! (Unless you know someone who was stranded on a island without citrus fruit, or a graduate student).

The take-home message is that our biology can run amuck when it isn't supplied with what it needs; and this is occurring much more frequently than we realize. In the nutrition section, we discussed how even sub-clinical deficiencies can lead to a problem, and here we would like to impress upon you that *physical activity is no exception!*

A big part of the problem is that most people are unaware because they have no measure of how little physical activity they are actually engaging in on a daily basis. We will delve further into this topic in the following pages. This may be particularly difficult to realize because many of us still feel busy. We work hard, have a lot of projects or interests and generally a lot going on. But for the average individual these days it's a different kind of work. The combination of a lack of physical activity with the added psycho-social stressors that we encounter in our current environment is in no uncertain terms a double whammy on our brain health.

The examples of deficiency discussed above also seem to produce fairly noticeable symptoms (goiters are hard to miss), however, the biological changes in response to PADS produces more subtle symptoms. You can't see or hear your arteries filling up with plaque, which is why heart disease has been termed the "silent killer." Luckily we don't wear our brains outside of the protective shell of our skulls, but if you've ever had the chance to see a brain that has been affected by Alzheimer's disease you'd be shocked by the physical difference when compared to a non-diseased brain. So even though it isn't as visible as a goiter, physical inactivity promotes a myriad of physiologically unfortunate situations.

Is It Really That Bad?

There are some disturbing data out there documenting just how inactive we are becoming. An interesting study came out a couple of years ago that analyzed databases maintained by each state in the United States. They didn't measure physical activity levels per se, but determined the behavioral patterns and occupations that people engaged in on a daily basis. Some of the highlights were a reported 71% decrease in the number of people commuting to work by walking and the 80% increase in the proportion of people working at a low physical activity type of occupation (i.e. desk job), when comparing the early 1950s to the year 2000. My, how times have changed! If you look at the worst combination of what this study described, it shows that 50-60 years ago, a lot of people walked to work on top of being physically active at work. Now it is probably more common for people to commute via vehicle to work and spend the day behind a computer "hammering" away on the keyboard.

Other studies have shown the importance of physical activity on decreasing the susceptibility to heart-disease, diabetes and cancer. In addition there is an ever strengthening link among these diseases to mood and cognitive disorders. To beat our point into the ground further, more and more scientific studies show the link between physical activity and improved mood and cognition. So in this case 2+2 does equal 4, and increased physical activity is essential to all aspects of our health, and subsequently our quality of life. What is starting to come to light is the vital importance of physical activity on brain health.

There are a couple things to consider. First, it is one thing to hear that you need to exercise more, but it is completely different if you have a measure of your activity. What does this mean? Well, you should measure your current activity so you know how you are doing. This was a task that we both tried a couple years ago, and quite honestly, we were shocked. We'll talk more about what we found, and what we decided to do about our activity levels. Second, you must realize that you should not view a physical activity routine as a short-term training program. You really must incorporate it into your lifestyle for any real benefit. Fortunately, some moderate changes can make a big difference, but they need to be a priority and you need to make it part of your life from here on out. Now it is never too late to change, and any positive change is good but it is our sincere hope that eventually most people will drive themselves to improve their physical capacity by starting this process sooner rather than later.

Balancing Act

There are several principles that you should keep in mind as you are making decisions about how to increase your levels of physical activity. As we mentioned above, "use it or lose it" is a real phenomenon that you should manage. You also should ask yourself, "what are my goals?" If you are happy with your current fitness level, then you will need to make decisions that are very different from someone who wants to increase his or her performance. Also, when we say you should prioritize physical activity, we don't mean that this should take precedence over everything in your life. Compulsive exercise can become a very serious problem, and you don't want to start down that road. But physical activity and exercise need to be given their due time. To step back even further, you should be cautious about spending too much time on any one aspect of your lifestyle, your efforts should always be focused around maintaining a balance that is optimal for you. So don't exercise so much that your efforts dedicated to sleep or mental activity suffer.

Overload Principle

As with many things, one of the best ways to improve is to challenge yourself. This is also true with exercise. The

Overload Principle is one of the basic tenants of exercise based on the idea of continually challenging one's self to improve performance. If you are able to walk at a 20 minute per mile pace, and you always walk the same route at the same pace you will maintain your performance level (barring injury) but you won't substantially increase your capacity to perform. In contrast, if you can walk at a pace of 20 minutes per mile on a given route, but challenge yourself by walking a few minutes at a pace of 15 minutes per mile or take a different route that has some hills, over time you will be able to increase your capacity for performance through challenging your body. The idea is that you need to carefully push your limits in order to increase your performance. Now this doesn't happen after one excursion, but by continually challenging yourself you can improve your performance. This concept of "overload" also carries over for mental activities as well as many other aspects of life. Truly, variety is the spice of life that allows us to live life more fully while becoming better prepared to deal with the obstacles that life throws our way.

Detraining & Atrophy: The Face Of UIOLI

While continually challenging ourselves is important to improve our capacity for performance, lack of training will rather quickly decrease our capacity for physical activity. Even maintenance training that is not sufficiently varied can cause problems like overuse injuries. Detraining is the loss of, or reduction in, biological mechanisms that allow us to perform at a given level. The frustrating, almost unfair, part of this is that it occurs very quickly. For example, a loss of up to 50% of an individual's aerobic capacity takes approximately 4 weeks. Now contrast this time-frame with the *3-6 months* it takes to increase your capacity to that level. This is an epic example of use it or lose it, and should drive home the point of prioritizing and making these changes part of your daily routine from here to eternity! Now you can recapture those gains, but it will take several months and it becomes a bit more difficult as we age, so the earlier we start and the better we are at maintaining our daily routine of physical activity the better off we'll be.

How Much is Too Much?

If a little bit of something is good for you, then a lot is better, right? Wrong. We discussed this point in the introductory chapter and we'll revisit it again here. Ninety-nine percent of the time you can get too much of a good thing. Exercise is no exception and you should be mindful of two things. The first is overtraining. Essentially, overtraining occurs when you exercise at too intense a level without sufficient rest for an extended period of time.

Overtraining will actually cause an individual's performance to suffer, so it is definitely something you need to be aware of. Physical activity or exercise is a very dynamic process that requires sufficient periods of rest so your body can repair itself. Although we're currently focusing on keeping our bodies active, as we'll discuss in subsequent chapters, rest is essential for our brains as well. For most people this won't be an issue because they probably don't have the time to train excessively. One of the tricks is to know when to work and when to rest. A key point to remember is that you don't want to take too much time off between workouts. In fact, light (lower intensity/shorter duration) workouts can actually help the biological repair process your body needs after more intense training helping to reduce soreness.

The second thing to avoid is unbalance in your priorities. As we mentioned above, you don't want to focus on one aspect of the program at the risk of neglecting another. Even if you're not exercising at a volume and frequency that will cause overtraining, you won't optimize the return on your efforts by just exercising without proper nutrition, rest and mental activity.

How To Approach Exercise (General And Age-Specific)

You've heard it before, but we'll say it again. Start slowly and listen to your body. No one knows your body better than you. You should also take the time to sit down and determine your goals. Once you know what you'd like to accomplish you can start to create a timeline and figure out the best way to achieve your goals, either on your own or with a fitness professional. In either case, check with your physician,

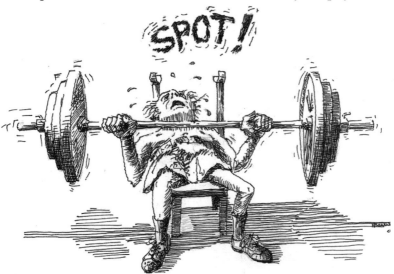

"Be sure to engage in age and fitness level appropriate exercise. Also, try to find a partner to exercise with that can 'spot' you when needed. You don't want to put yourself at risk for injury."

especially if you have ever been diagnosed with any major medical issues. One thing you need to start thinking is that this is now your way of life. It can't be thought of as a finite diet or exercise campaign to drop some pounds, this is an ongoing way of life that will keep you functioning optimally. We'll have some specific suggestions at the end of this section on how to measure your current status, and implement some changes in your physical activity to help you make this a part of your daily life.

Making The Path Of Least Resistance Less Traveled

Many things are convenient and easy these days, particularly in terms of our daily physical demands. You should develop the mindset that it is the journey as much as the destination that is important. That our effort, our blood, our sacrifice, our commitment, contribute more to our person than the outcome those efforts are directed towards.

In many cases, we seek to find the path of least resistance. This is an underlying theme in nature, an instinct. We can see this when we watch water flow downhill. However, there are instances and situations when it can be too easy, too convenient. That is where we are now. The changes that we have experienced over the past 50-100 years have vastly improved our daily way-of-life, but they have also brought on a new set of problems. In many ways we need to make a conscious effort to make the path of least resistance the path least traveled.

Moving On

There are two points in our journey that will be pinnacle. The first being, what do we need? The second is how do we maintain our approach to filling that need? These are lifestyle choices. One of our main goals will be to improve the way you live for the rest of your life. This requires addressing the two pinnacle questions. In the following chapters, we will discover how physical activity and exercise can help us achieve our goals of brain fitness. It's a pretty tall order. You might even feel a little anxious about it, but exercise can help anxiety too. Let's find out how.

Neural Nugget #3 – Oxygen For Exercise, Or Not

As most people know, there are two 'kinds' of exercise, aerobic and anaerobic. The distinction between the two concerns the use of oxygen to produce energy that our muscles use to move: aerobic (with oxygen), anaerobic (without oxygen). We will try our best to keep this nugget as light on the biochemistry as possible, but we need to think in very general biochemical terms for a minute.

The main concept is that the type of metabolism that our muscles employ depends on the intensity of the exercise. Very intense exercise that lasts for a relatively short time requires energy very quickly and therefore relies almost entirely on anaerobic metabolism. This type of intense brief exercise is anaerobic. Examples of anaerobic exercise include sprinting and weight lifting.

In contrast, less intense, usually prolonged exercise that uses oxygen to produce energy is termed, aerobic. Low to moderate intensity jogging/running, biking, and swimming fall into the category of aerobic exercise.

It should be noted that many sports and activities fall somewhere between these metabolic definitions of exercise since they incorporate varying intensities that require muscle to work in both aerobic and anaerobic condition

Now you may be wondering, "Are weights any good for my noggin?" That's a great question. When people talk about the benefits of exercise on health, nine times out of ten the discussion will focus on aerobic exercise. So we need to ask ourselves, is anaerobic exercise beneficial to brain health? And, if so, why should we bother since we already know that aerobic exercise is good for brain health?

Research continues to demonstrate the benefits of moderate or reasonably intense weight training to improve emotional and cognitive function. Studies show that weight training (anaerobic exercise) has positive effects on mood, attention, and short-term memory compared to individuals in control groups who had weekly warm-up and stretch sessions. This data also indicates that there is more to it than getting together with people (social aspects). At least part of the benefit is due to anaerobic exercise.

But why bother with weights? We want to remind you that you should strive for a balanced approach to fitness. Exercise routines should incorporate both endurance (aerobic) and strength (anaerobic) training. We're not talking about blood vessel poppin', t-shirt rippin' workouts; light to moderate, multi-repetition weight training works, too. You can obtain many other health benefits from weight training that will supplement your aerobic routines. Here are several to consider:

1) *Weight training builds muscle mass. Now unless you get really, really serious about weight training you won't have to worry about looking like Mr. Universe. That said, increases in muscle mass help increase our overall metabolism....even at rest, which means pound-for-pound we can burn more calories.*

2) *Weight training helps strengthen bones. The load placed on our bones during weight training causes our bones to respond by increasing their density and thickness. Maintaining strong bones is an especially important benefit for women to help ward off osteoporosis. It's also very important for people as they age. Falls are not uncommon and broken bones from falls in elderly individuals can be debilitating and very difficult to recover from.*

3) *Multi-joint weight training exercises (like squats or lunges) help improve balance and coordination. Again, this has obvious benefits for people as they age. Stronger muscles and better balance clearly make it more likely you can recover from a stumble before it turns into a fall. And let's be honest, who among us couldn't use a little more coordination?*

A couple of words of caution:

1) *Always talk with your physician to determine what kinds of exercise are safe for you before you start an exercise program or make drastic changes to your current program.*
2) *Get advice from a professional. There are many personal trainers available to help you get started with weight training. Look for someone certified by a reputable institution. The American College of Sports Medicine, and the National Strength and Conditioning Association are two examples.*
3) *Start slowly, and listen to your body. This is especially important if you haven't been active for a while. Remember that through exercise, in addition to helping your brain, you are re-sculpting your body so it is natural to be a little sore. But, overdoing it can make you so sore that you miss your next workout, or even worse cause an injury.*
4) *Lift with a partner. It is always a good idea to have someone there to "spot" you when you are lifting. Having a spotter will help you stay motivated and committed, but is also a very important safety measure, especially when working with heavy weights.*

So, check with your doc, start slow, and get pumped up...for your general health and your mental health!

CHAPTER 7

MOVING FEELINGS

Exercising Control Over Your Emotions

"A vigorous five-mile walk will do more good for an unhappy but otherwise healthy adult than all the medicine and psychology in the world."
- Paul Dudley White (physician and cardiologist)

Emotions are funny things. They're not always logical or appropriate, they don't always serve a positive end and sometimes they can get us in a lot of trouble if not held in check. They also influence much of what people think of us. They frame who we are, and become a subtle, or not so subtle, backdrop on which we build our memories.

Exercise For Mind, Body And Mood

Exercise improves mood. A lot of research has investigated changes in mood following a single-session in almost any group of people imaginable. In the majority of cases, when test subjects exercise at a moderate intensity and duration, mood improves. People often want to know what type of exercise (aerobic or anaerobic) is "best." The answer is...both. Both aerobic and anaerobic exercise result in elevated mood, and both have distinct advantages in terms of how they affect our bodies. A comparison of these two types of exercise is provided in the *Neural Nugget #3, Oxygen for*

Exercise, or Not. There are many ways to incorporate both types of exercise into your normal routine, but if you're new to the exercise scene, a good way to work on both, plus your balance is by trying Tai Chi or Yoga. In fact, Tai Chi and Yoga are two exercises that have the ability to combine "below-the-neck" benefits of aerobic *and* anaerobic exercise, while simultaneously focusing on stress reduction; and both consistently improve mood.

How Long Will This Take?

Some of the changes that occur with exercise take several weeks, particularly if you are looking for a difference in appearance or a change in your blood pressure. But for mood, there is good news! There are many studies showing that you can start to reap the benefits of improving emotional intelligence immediately with a single session of exercise. Putting in the time to exercise *consistently* has added benefit. A study by Hoffman and Hoffman in 2008 reported that middle-aged individuals who exercised regularly showed larger improvements in mood after a single exercise session compared to people who never exercise. To be clear, the individuals who never exercise did show improved mood after the single session, however, it wasn't as large as the improvement in mood experienced by the group that exercised on a regular basis.

This speaks to the importance of making exercise a priority and part of your normal routine. If you can engage in regular exercise, you'll get more bang for your buck from a single session. It's similar to compound interest, as you put more in, your returns on investment (ROI) roll back into your account causing your subsequent return on investment to increase. And like any financial advisor will tell you, it's never too late to start. Remember that in these studies, even the people who never exercised experienced improvements in mood. So anyone just starting out should get some benefit, and with time, their investment in regular physical activity will start to produce more substantial returns in terms of positive mood. This is a beautiful example of an upward spiral, these are difficult to start and take effort to maintain, but they get easier and easier as you go. Start to build your emotional reserve now! You never know when you may need it.

Exercise In The Battle Against Mood Disorders

Is there any potential for exercise to help people with mood disorders? Research on the subject is positive and shows that exercise is beneficial for people with depression and/or anxiety. Exercise can help in a couple of different ways. First, exercise can decrease your odds of developing depression, and reduce the severity of depressive symptoms in people with depression. Second, it can help antidepressant drugs work better. We're not saying that exercise is a cure for depression, and there are many people who are helped by taking antidepressant medications. However, by the same argument, drugs are not a cure for depression either.

Dealing With Depression

The effectiveness of exercise as a prevention or treatment for depression has been gaining scientific support for over a decade now. It has the potential to serve as part of a prevention strategy, along with other lifestyle choices, to reduce the risk of developing depression. Further, it is effective in elevating mood in non-depressed people and can reduce the feelings of depression in people with depressive disorders. It also has the ability to serve as an adjunctive, or add-on therapy, especially in treatment resistant cases of depression .

Running Down The Risk

Studies show that exercise decreases the risk for developing depression in adults, fifty to ninety plus years old. This effect in older adults is important to consider because having an emotional disorder increases your risk for developing a cognitive disorder, and vice versa. Exercise and increased physical activity are effective in decreasing the severity of these diseases, which will be exceedingly important if an individual is suffering from other health problems as well.

Running Up Recovery

Other studies show exercise is effective in treating depression in individual's suffering from neurodegenerative disease. Alzheimer's disease patients who were also depressed showed an improvement in mood with 3 months of exercise, whereas control subjects actually got worse over the 3 month period. As we discuss in chapter 9, exercise is an effective strategy for preventing or improving the symptoms of Alzheimer's disease. Losing your memory is a frightening prospect, and it probably isn't surprising that cognitive decline would get people down, if not precipitate depression. Luckily, we can attack both the mood and memory decline by working on all four pillars of brain fitness, and exercise is a crucial component.

In fact, there is evidence that exercise is as effective a treatment for depression as antidepressant drugs. A very important point is that exercise can be effective in reducing feelings of depression in people who don't respond to drug treatment. Studies show individuals that don't respond to drug treatment alone have decreased depressive symptoms when physicians combine their drug therapies with exercise. Importantly, both aerobic and non-aerobic forms of exercise seem to work well at treating depression. So whether you'd rather play tennis or lift weights, your mood will benefit either way.

So why isn't that a standard-issue treatment for depression? Why don't doctors prescribe a run around the block for everyone with depression? Although that would likely benefit the patient, there are several factors standing in the way. First, people with depression are depressed. Sounds obvious, but this is a major health issue to deal with. People with depression can find it impossible to get out of bed for days, potentially weeks. This might put a damper on their ability to head out for a jog. In many cases depression also has a variety of somatic symptoms (or bodily sensations), including altered appetite, extreme fatigue and pain. These are some substantial obstacles to overcome. One way to attack these issues is with support, with friends, family, or anyone in your social network. Our support network is powerful and may be the spark to get us moving, or the measure of accountability that will keep us going through tough times. As we've already discussed, the benefits can be immediate. Sometimes just taking those first steps is the toughest part of the battle.

Dosing Up

The amount of exercise you do will influence the return that you get. Again, kind of like our banking example. You'll earn interest on whatever you save, but you'll get more interest back if you make a bigger deposit. This is a neat aspect of exercise, that it has a dose-response relationship with mood.

Scientists use the term "dose-response" to describe how varying doses of a drug or medication will influence what you're looking at (i.e. mood, blood pressure, blood sugar levels, etc.). A larger dose of drug usually leads to bigger the change in mood, to a point. With a little exercise, say 10 minutes of walking, you get a little reduction in the symptoms of depression. With some more exercise, say 20 minutes of brisk walking, you will have a larger reduction the symptoms of depression. We want to make clear that in almost every case (exercise included), this relationship of "more is better" only holds true up to a certain amount of drug or exercise. As we discussed in the introduction, too much of anything and you may fall out of balance to a point where bad things can happen.

What would be even better is to avoid a disease like depression all together. This is an instance where it might help to think of exercise as a vitamin (although some of us would argue that we should view it the other way around, vitamins are like exercise). Again, we're not saying that exercise will prevent depression, but it has the ability to decrease your odds of developing depression, by helping to put more into your *BrainFit* reserve account.

Boosting Drug Treatment

Treating depression is tricky to start with, and if a person's depression doesn't respond to a specific drug, doctors may try another dose of the same drug, a different drug, or a combination of more than one antidepressant. Sometimes people and physicians get lucky and find an effective treatment the first time. Other times (about 40%), it can take a lot of trial and error to a find an effective treatment and there are many cases where individuals don't satisfactorily respond to any drugs at all. This is another opportunity where exercise can often help. Exercise has proven potential for use as an adjunctive or additional therapy for depression. It can increase a person's ability to respond to antidepressant drugs when they are not responding to drugs alone, providing physicians with more tools to manage mood disorders.

You should always check with your physician before making major changes in your physical activity, especially if you are already under treatment for something, to be sure that you won't injure yourself. Some medications can actually influence your *ability* to exercise or your body's response to exercise. For example, beta-blockers given to people to help manage heart disease will limit the maximal heart rate that can be achieved during exercise. This is a good thing if you're heart is beating too fast when you are just sitting around, but it might be impossible to reach the estimated target heart-rate for your age. Other types of drugs can alter perception, coordination, and balance. If the label warns you not to operate 'heavy machinery' after you have taken it, you probably shouldn't go rock-climbing either.

Attacking Anxiety

Anxiety disorders are both common and debilitating. Exercise can reduce anxiety after a single session. It appears that both aerobic and anaerobic types of exercise have the ability to improve feelings of anxiety. How this works isn't exactly clear. It may be related to an opportunity to release pent-up frustrations (positive use of excess energy) like we discuss later in this chapter. It may also be related to the chemicals that our brains release during exercise, like dopamine or endorphins (our body's self-made morphine) that helps to relax. No matter how it works, it works and we should be willing to use it.

Another intriguing possibility is that, for people with an anxiety disorder, exercise may provide the opportunity to have control over some of the feelings they have during an anxiety-attack. Studies show that individuals with generalized anxiety disorder experience lower levels of anxiety after a session of aerobic or resistance type training. Interestingly, both exercise and panic attacks activate parts of the sympathetic nervous system. These include increased heart rate and blood pressure, flushing and sweating, increased rate of breathing, and so on. The idea is that because exercise exposes people to many of the same sensations they feel during a panic attack they become familiar with them and aware of their control over them. They can regulate how often and how hard they exercise, ultimately allowing them to exert control over sensations that arise from a subconscious cue during a panic attack. The idea of control is very important for both depression and anxiety disorders as is the ability to effectively cope with stress.

Coping With Stress

Many people view stress as a psychological state conjured up by annoyances that life brings our way. Situations at work, home, or major life events (chronic illness of a family member) can certainly be sources of stress. For some time now, researchers have adapted a much broader definition of stress, and it would serve us all well to begin to think along these lines. For a deeper look at stress, you can read *Neural Nugget #4, Stressing Out*. In a very broad sense, stress is the disruption of physiological balance (eustasis). Anything that alters your balanced state is a stressor that your body and your mind must attend to in order to return you to balance. You rely on your physical balance to stand and walk without falling over. You don't really have to think about that, because you 'practice' it every day just by getting up and moving around. Other parts of your life require balance as well and sometimes they are not quite so automatic.

Many psychological or physical stressors can throw your system out of balance. Psychological stress includes things like an impending deadline at work with the boss breathing down your neck for results. Physical stress can be having the flu or being hungry, or even too full. All of these throw your body out of balance and initiate your 'stress response' in an attempt to return to a balanced state. You've altered your 'balance' in a way that requires your body and brain to respond.

Some of these situations are more obvious. Having the flu is hard to miss, since your body has to mount an immune response to fight off a virus. Other situations are more subtle. The concept of eating as a stressor might be a little more novel for most people. Let's say you just ate a nice big hamburger. In this situation, once you've ingested food, your stomach needs to break it down both chemically and mechanically. Once broken down into the more basic components of your meal (proteins, carbohydrates, fats), your stomach absorbs the nutrients and transports them to various parts of your body through your blood stream. Various organs in your body (including your brain) recognize the increased levels of fat, carbohydrate and protein in your blood and evoke other hormonal responses to help you store or burn this newfound energy. The point being that eating changes the internal state of your body and your body responds to this change to bring you back towards a balance point.

So using this broad definition, you can have both 'good' and 'bad' forms of stress. Exercise, as long as it doesn't cause injury and isn't excessive or compulsive, should be viewed as a good stress. It evokes internal biological states that your body responds to. Now your body is smart, when you exercise regularly for an extended period of time your body begins to adapt so that you work more efficiently the next time you exercise. What's interesting is many of these adaptations that make your body more efficient in dealing with good exercise stress, may also provide you with the tools to more effectively deal with other stressors, or at least the disruption of our internal biology and psychology caused by these stressors.

The Good, The Bad And The Ugly

We won't dive into the ugly this go around, but we will take a look at good and bad stress. Bad stress is an ever present obstacle in our high-paced society. Unfortunately, for many of us, in the battle between good and bad, bad is winning. Because the bad stress is coming out on top more often than not, it has more of an opportunity to run rampant, particularly for the vast majority of people whose physical demands of daily routines are minimal to non-existent. Remember, the difference in physical requirements for the average working individual has changed drastically in the last 50-100 years. Now this in and of itself may not have posed too much of a burden, but in addition to our dwindling physical activity the average person's exposure to stress has increased as physical activity has decreased. So we've experienced a decline in a good stress and an increase in bad stress, not the balance we're looking for.

Exercise: A Good Stress Or A Bad Stress?

Let's imagine for a minute that a wicked witch with green skin and a big pointy nose who's full of anger because someone dropped a house on her sister, represents bad stress.

Let's also imagine that a leotard-clad, good witch named Glinda represents exercise (good stress). Glinda has a very calming and settling effect when she shows up to comfort the confused Dorothy who was just implicated in killing a witch who she'd never even met before. Her presence essentially shooed away the wicked witch (bad stress). In fact, Glinda was so calming that even the little people came out after all those years of oppression under the stressed out wicked witch of the East. Back to our point. Exercise is a good-stress that reduces bad-stress. Exercise is the Glinda to your wicked witches of the West. Generally, people feel that their stress levels decline

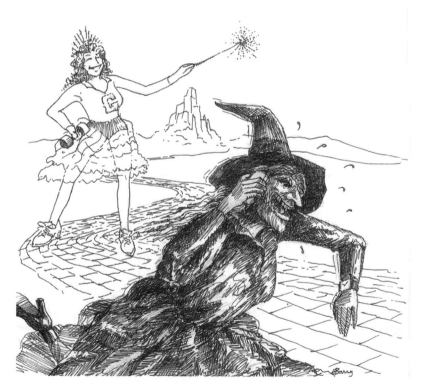

"'Good Stress Glinda has the ability to help us deal with and ward-off those ugly bad stressors brought to us by the 'Wicked Stressed Witch of the West'."

when they exercise regularly, or even after a single session. These effects likely occur in a couple of different ways.

First, exercise reduces *perceived* stress levels. This appears to be a short-term effect related to a recent bout of exercise. Things just don't bother you as much right after you've been out sweating. That pile of laundry and those dishes in the sink just don't get to you as much as they normally might, for a short while anyway. However, if you make exercise a part of your regular routine, the additive effect of daily exercise may produce a more consistent stress reduction for you.

Second, exercise acts as a means to reduce your responsiveness to stressful events. Although there is still some debate on the topic, exercise may have the ability to prepare your body and your brain to better handle other day-to-day stressors that you encounter. Academic types call this idea *cross-stressor adaptation*, meaning that by building your ability to handle the stress of exercise, you build your ability to handle stress in general. Whether or not exercise ultimately proves to provide a true cross-stressor adaptation by way of reduced activation of our stress response is still unclear. However, it does offer the opportunity for your body to better prepare for a challenge. There is evidence that exercise changes the responsivity of your hypothalamic-pituitary-adrenal (HPA) axis, which is one of the main drivers of your stress system. Although dysfunction can happen at several levels of the HPA axis, exercise has the ability to help you view stressful situations as less stressful *and* change your body's hormonal response to stress. This, in turn, will feedback to influence your perception of stress as well. This is clearly a win-win situation.

So as you work through your self-assessment you should consider the type of stress that you have in your life (i.e. good or bad). Then you can determine the control that you have over the situation, and the amount of time that you're exposed to the stressor. Being aware of what type of stressor you're dealing with will help you recognize particular problem areas and develop a strategy to bring yourself back toward balance.

Energy Balance

Personally We like to think of exercise as a positive way to burn-off energy. If you've ever watched Cesar Milan's program, *The Dog Whisperer*, you realize that the ability of exercise to reduce extra 'nervous energy' is pretty amazing. In many ways it should be unsettling for us to have to sit behind a computer at a desk most of the day for a substantial chunk of our life. That isn't the way we have lived for the majority of time that the human species has walked this planet. We have energy to burn. When we don't use it, it accumulates in several ways. One is physically, as fat. Another way this pent up energy can manifest itself is in behavioral terms. This is why it is amazing that schools have actually eliminated physical education classes. It seems crazy to ask school aged children to sit still for most of a 6-hour day. Beyond the difficult requirement of asking kids to sit still for that long, we should be ensuring they we expose them to at least the minimal level of physical activity, thereby promoting health benefits. If nothing else at least wear the kids out for the first 45 minutes of the day to take some of the heat off the teachers.

In the realm of 'mental energy', you have to think about what you're asking your brain to do. As was discussed earlier in the book, our brains are energy hogs. This 3 pound organ that sits in our heads uses up to 20% of the energy and oxygen that we take in. There are many, many, many distinct regions of the brain. These regions 'talk' to each other via various connections (similar to the electrical wiring you'd find in a building), but which regions are talking, and how loudly they are talking is very dependent upon what our current activity is.

If you're writing papers, or crunching numbers or filling out reports all day long you're using very specific areas of your brain. Granted it will require many brain regions to perform these tasks, but it ends up being the same type of task. One thing that exercise can do is allow your brain to expend energy while performing a different task. This will still include some of the brain regions you're using while sitting at your desk, but will also require the involvement of other regions that arc uscd much lcss when we are sedentary. All of this leads to less pent up energy and healthier behavioral responses to stress

Escape From Sedentary Island To Exercise Peninsula

If you're too young, or just didn't tune in, *Cheers* was a comedy on television back in the 1980's centered around a group of Bostonian bar patrons. Many people can easily relate to this extremely funny show with a very catchy theme song. The opening lines of the theme song spoke to the role that bad-stress could play in one's life and the way that the bar served as an escape from that stress. It illustrated the need for people to get away from the stress in their daily lives, to escape and be in a place where 'everybody knows your name'. Now a few frosty 'barley pops' would likely help you attain your goal of escaping your daily stress and may be a great choice for some people if they indulge in moderation (this is starting to sound like a beer commercial). But there are some better choices that won't increase your risk of alcoholism.

Exercise can be a great way to escape from the immediate pressures of the everyday world. It can provide relative solitude if you put on your headphones and go for a long walk. It can also serve as a social escape, especially if you meet with people to work out, or get together with other people who are training for a common event. Now contrast this with the habit of plopping down in front of the TV for several hours when you get home, or meeting up at the bar for a couple drinks after work. I'm not saying you can't or shouldn't do those things, but they should be the exception, not the rule. We all have our vices and we're not asking you to give them up completely. We just want you to find balance in your life to enjoy the 'good' stressors so you can offset the 'bad' ones.

Moving On

In this chapter we highlighted the importance of exercise for general emotional health and the potential that exercise holds as a preventative measure and a treatment for mood disorders. One of the key concepts is that we need to start early to build up our reserve in case we need to draw from that bank account someday. But if we do build up this reserve, this *BrainFit* bank account, how and when will we spend it?

Let's find out.

CHAPTER 8

WORKING YOUR BRAINS OFF

Exercise For Your Mind-Body Interactions

"Genius may have its limitations, but stupidity is not thus handicapped."
   -   Elbert Hubbard, circa 1900 (writer, artist and philosopher)

Traditionally, we thought that exercise was mainly good for your bones, muscles, and heart. So we wouldn't be true to our Neuroscience roots if we didn't prattle on, at least a little bit, about the less publicized changes occurring in the brain. In fact, many profound bits of scientific evidence about how exercise affects the physical structure of our brain has begun to accumulate in the last several years. How does exercise benefit the physical health of the brain? The answer isn't simple and there are many smart individuals still figuring that out. So far, exercise appears to alter the brain by several means. But one thing is for sure, the brain responds to exercise, and almost always in a good way.

Some of the most exciting neuroscience research suggests that working our muscles actually changes the structure of our brain! One of the most exciting effects of exercise is neurogenesis (the birth of new neurons), which has been shown in rodents and non-human primates. Although this hasn't been shown in humans directly, (due to technical and ethical reasons) it seems highly probable. This is very exciting for health care practitioners and researchers seeking insight into how new neurons are born. Ultimately, understanding more about this process will lead to better treatments for neurodegenerative diseases.

Another exciting component of exercise effects on the brain is the increase in levels of proteins called growth factors. You can think of these proteins as "fertilizer for the brain." To date these haven't received the same amount of press as neurogenesis, but they are starting to get more air time. One that you may have heard of in the media is Brain Derived Neurotrophic Factor, commonly identified by the acronym BDNF. This is an interesting molecule that increases with exercise and, intriguingly, with antidepressant drugs. In fact, increases in BDNF appear to be critical for antidepressant drugs to work. This means that exercise and antidepressants may be working through the same mechanism, at least partially. However, one of them doesn't carry nearly as many adverse side effects as the other. You can guess which.

In lab animals, BDNF also increases when researchers add complexity (enrichment) to an animal's environment. Typically, rats live in boring cages but if you give them things to explore, like toys, BDNF in their brains increases. The reason why BDNF increases are so exciting is that it helps increase synaptic connections (the connections between brain cells) and neuron growth. This means if you can do things that increase BDNF in a controlled way, like exercise, you can give your brain the fertilizer it needs for new brain cell growth and connectivity.

A couple of other growth factors you will probably hear about in the near future from the popular media will be Vascular-Endothelial Growth Factor (VEGF) and Insulin-Like Growth Factor-1 (IGF-1). These growth factors have well documented roles in the growth of new blood vessels. Since the brain is such an energy hog and doesn't maintain any

appreciable amount of stored energy the network of blood
vessels that feed it and remove waste products is absolutely
critical. Because exercise increases these growth factors you
can use it to help fertilize your neurovascular system as well.
Furthermore, these growth factors may play a role in the
growth and stability of the connections between nerve cells.

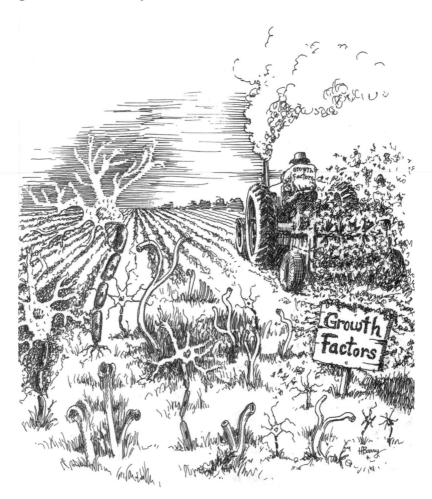

*"Growth factors are fertilizer for the brain.
Spreading them around the 'neuron farm' will help neurons
grow. Exercise helps your brain spread the fertilizer."*

We'll talk more about this in the upcoming section on synaptic strength.

Exercise also has well documented effects on growth hormone, and an array of other hormones that regulate energy storage and release. A review of all of these is beyond the scope of this book but we wanted to point out a few of the key research findings to help you understand the positive benefits at work in your noggin' while you're out there pounding the pavement.

Synchronizing Synaptic Strength

When we talk about synapses, we are referring to a contact point or connection between two nerve cells (neurons). We'll also spend some more time on this in chapters 10 and 13 in the context of mental exercise. Just to clarify, nerve cells don't actually touch each other in most cases, but they come really close. The space between neurons as they come close to each other, called synapses, allows them to send chemicals from one brain cell to the other. This is one major way that cells in the brain communicate.

The brain is in a constant state of flux. Nerve cells send out projections and sometimes they become permanent. Sometimes those projections never really settle and are pruned back. But when a significant connection is made it's important that it becomes stable and efficient at transmitting its message. Growth factors aid in the processes by which nerve cells "feel out" new connections and strengthen connections once they are made. So exercise, by increasing growth factors, can increase the likelihood that new synapses between neurons stabilize.

To recap, exercise increases synaptic strength on two fronts. First, you can improve your performance through repetition and practice. You strengthen connections between neurons involved in controlling a behavior with repetitive exercise because you give those neurons more opportunities to connect. This increases the odds those connections will stabilize, allowing you to more effectively execute that exercise behavior in the future. Second, you create conditions for those connections to become permanent. As we just discussed, exercise increases the release of several growth factors, including BDNF, VEGF, and IGF-1, which help fertilize neurons, synapses and your brain's blood supply. Taken together, these effects of exercise provide a more 'fertile field' for growth and connectivity.

Boosting Brain Metabolism

Remember that our brains tend to be energy hogs. They consume a disproportionate amount of oxygen and nutrients for their relative weight in the body. Further, these processes are closely guarded. Whereas other muscles or organs that are not directly involved in exercise experience a reduced flow of blood during exercise (a phenomenon known as the exercise-shunt due to the redirection of blood away from less-active organs to working muscle), the brain maintains or slightly increases its consumption of oxygen, nutrients and blood flow. Although you might think that the brain is just sitting up in your skull while you walk or jog, along for the ride so to speak, it is actually reacting. It is anticipating and controlling many processes that are happening in your body while you exercise, and even more so if you are in an interactive environment like a sport where you need to constantly predict and react to the game. So while it's good to start walking, a great goal would be to end up in a racket-ball court with one of those little blue balls zooming past your head at 50 mph; that will keep your brain busy and reactions sharp!

Really, what you are doing with exercise is improving the overall biological environment that your brain experiences within your body. Increased ability of your body to transport more oxygen or nutrients with less effort is an enormous benefit to your brain. Not only does this improve performance, but it reduces the energy required to deal with stress, since your delivery mechanisms have become more efficient. Other important adaptations include the ability to handle biological by-products (waste products) that your brain needs to get rid of on a regular basis.

Substantial research exists documenting the beneficial effects of physical activity and exercise on several other aspects of your biology. Cardiovascular exercise can improve our circulatory system, the vascular-interstate through which our blood travels delivering oxygen, nutrients, and hormones to your organs and cells. Exercise improves this network of thoroughfares by paving new routes, increasing the volume of traffic, all while optimizing the efficiency of the system. Exercise can promote vascularization in many organs including the heart and brain.

Although research on the effects of exercise on increasing vascularization of the brain is a burgeoning field, it will likely prove to be a substantial contributor to our understanding of brain health. Related to this, a recent large study by Dr. Thomas Montine from the University of Washington, reports that 33% of the risk of dementia stems from disease of small blood-vessels in the brain. In this 12-year study, 3,400 men and women over age 65 volunteered for periodic cognitive testing and a brain autopsy upon their death. In the 221 autopsies performed, researchers discovered that small blood vessel disease accounted for about 1/3 of the risk for dementia. This type of small blood vessel disease may not be noticed; in contrast to what we typically associate with vascular disease, for example, a stroke or clot blocking a larger vessel. But over time these effects are likely to add up and result in cognitive impairment. So this is a substantial number, if 1 out of 3 cases of dementia are attributable to vessel disease in the brain, then taking better care of our neurovascular system will help reduce the risk of acquiring this subcategory of dementia. Exercise will help you do this.

Aerobic exercise also increases blood volume, allowing the body to carry larger quantities of oxygen and nutrients to working organs, while removing metabolic by-products. Increased blood-volume also allows for better control of body temperature and allows us to handle longer durations of exercise/physical activity before dehydration begins to set in.

The effects of cardiovascular exercise on the heart have been extensively documented. It increases ventricular chamber size, contractility, and volume of blood pumped per heart beat, which combine to increase the efficiency at which the heart can work. These changes to our peripheral cardiovascular system are also important for our brains. Since the brain controls all the rest of the organs in the body a more efficient cardiovascular system will require less input from the brain. It's kind of like power steering. If you (the brain) are driving a car (the body) without power steering (the cardiovascular system) it takes a lot of effort to turn the wheel, but with power steering, you can make small adjustments that the steering mechanism will respond to. Similarly, in people with good cardiovascular fitness, the heart needs to beat fewer times to supply the body with the same amount of blood.

It is important to note these "below the neck effects" because of the strong mind-body link that we mentioned earlier in this section. Our bodies provide the environment for our brain, and our brain helps control our bodies to optimize how we function. It's a give and take relationship, and your brain and body are stuck as partners for life, so you may as well do whatever you can to help them get along.

Related to this partnership is the effect of exercise on how our brain regulates many of the processes in the body that are automated. The autonomic nervous system takes care of many of the day-to-day functions that need to be done, but we don't need, or want, to think about. This part of the nervous system controls heart-rate, breathing, blood pressure, and changes in the levels of hormones within our bodies. Exercise improves autonomic function, which may play into some of the benefits of exercise on stress, which we discussed in the last chapter. Exercise also influences a number of hormonal systems. For example, exercise has very important affects on how our bodies recognize insulin. As we discussed in chapter 4, the better your body is at responding to insulin, the better off your overall metabolism will work. Losing response to insulin is a big step toward diabetes. Exactly how all this happens is still a matter of intense research, but if you look at the 35,000-foot view, it will be obvious that exercise & physical activity improve your body's function, which intimately helps out your brain as well.

Perfect Practice Makes Perfect

A favorite response of coaches everywhere whenever someone utters "practice makes perfect" will be that "perfect practice makes perfect." This means that if you practice something incorrectly, you will learn to execute it incorrectly, so in reality practice may not make perfect. In fact, practice may make you perfectly incorrect. This is a good concept to keep in mind as we start to plan how we want to live. If we're going to take the time to do something we may as well do it right from the start. We want to avoid the mindset of, "There's never enough time to do something right the first time around, but there always seems to be enough time to do it again."

Making The Conscious Unconscious

As we've just discussed, many of the things your brain does for you are already automatic. You don't have to remember to tell your heart to beat, or your eyes to blink or your diaphragm to contract so you breathe. But, if you want to, you can think about those functions and control, or at least influence them. This concept is relevant to our next point, which is to make the conscious unconscious. If you could make things "automatic" or "reflexive" so you didn't have to think about them, imagine how much time you could free up to think about other things.

Relative to this concept, let's explore different kinds of memory for a minute. Declarative memory is the kind of memory that you can verbalize or tell someone else about. This includes memories about your childhood, how we get from your house to the supermarket, battling that fish that got away, and so on. Implicit memory is the kind of memory that you know, but might not realize you know. This includes things like throwing a ball, riding a bike, walking (and potentially chewing gum at the same time), or brushing your teeth. We have done these actions so many times that we can perform them without devoting much, if any, of our attention to them. They're also sometimes difficult to verbalize. You can't just tell someone how to ride a bike.

The interesting thing is that implicit memories generally start out requiring a lot of our attention and focus. But as we practice and master them, they become second nature. Most people don't have to spend a lot of time thinking about how to walk. But watch a seven-month-old sometime. It consumes their attention. And when they lose focus, splat! But after some practice, and some falls, they are able to walk successfully and start to do other things at the same time. Look around, talk, chase the dog, draw on the walls, etc.

Another interesting point to think about is implicit memories are not that drastically affected by aging or Alzheimer's. Now it may not matter to you whether or not you can type once you have Alzheimer's, which is why it is important to engage in learning new things that require focus and attention. Once you master a skill you need to venture back into the realm of the apprentice.

Reducing Diabetes

The role of exercise in preventing or managing diabetes may be one of the most dramatic ways in which exercise can help stave off disease, including cognitive decline. Diabetes is associated with a score of other diseases. Whether or not it directly causes other specific diseases is inconsequential. There are plenty of data showing that diabetes increases the risk for, and worsens the outcome of several other types of disease.

Controlling blood sugar levels is a very serious game for diabetics, so careful implementation of any exercise program must involve a physician. Evidence continues to accumulate illuminating the deleterious effect of diabetes on brain function. Not only does it affect how energy management systems function it also influences people's ability to learn and remember.

One form of diabetes occurs when the body (pancreas) stops producing the hormone, insulin. In the other form of diabetes, the body has become insensitive to insulin, that is the pancreas is making insulin, but organs in the body don't recognize it all that well. Insulin is responsible for helping bring glucose into the cells of the body from the blood stream. As we alluded to in the above discussion on growth factors, one of the big benefits of exercise for diabetics is that it increases sensitivity to insulin.

Peripheral neuropathy is a condition that can occur in diabetes where the nerves innervating the body's extremities began to retract. This can lead to feelings of numbness in the hands and feet. Once the nerves begin to deteriorate, this elevates the risk for secondary injuries. For diabetic individuals, who will also have problems with circulation in their limbs, the loss of sensation caused by peripheral neuropathy can cause additional problems. What can, and often does, happen is a small injury may occur on the foot, which goes unnoticed since the person can't feel it. Since they are unaware that the injury exists, they don't tend to it and it can become infected. These types of infections can become very serious and can potentially require amputation of the limb if they are not addressed quickly. Therefore, although exercise is highly beneficial for diabetics, they must use it cautiously.

There are currently no definitive treatments for diabetic peripheral neuropathy. However, exercise decreases the risk of developing the symptoms of peripheral neuropathy. In a 4-year longitudinal study, investigators examined how 4 hours of treadmill exercise per week reduced the development of neuropathy in diabetic patients. Over the course of the study, the number of diabetic patients that developed symptoms of peripheral neuropathy was substantially lower when the individuals exercised. None of the exercising diabetic individuals developed motor neuropathy, while approximately 17% (almost 1 in 5 people) of the non-exercising group developed the symptom. Further, only 6% of exercising diabetics developed sensory neuropathy during the course of the 4-year study, while approximately 30% of non-exercising diabetics developed this symptom. This is a huge improvement in stopping sensory neuropathy, which is important, because the lack of sensation (numbness) that is associated with this symptom is often what leads to diabetic ulcers on the feet. As we mentioned above, these ulcers can become infected and gangrenous ultimately requiring amputation of a limb; or if the infection isn't caught, death. In fact, diabetic peripheral neuropathy is a leading cause of non-traumatic foot amputation. So if you're diabetic, and you've grown attached to your feet be sure to use them or you'll be at substantially increased odds of losing them.

In people who have previously suffered from foot ulcers, weight bearing exercise showed a decreased risk of re-ulceration with increased levels of weight-bearing activity. So those who had the highest levels of weight-bearing activity throughout the day had the lowest risk of re-ulceration compared to the group with the lowest level of weight-bearing exercise. Even individuals performing moderate levels of weight-bearing activity were at reduced risk compared to the low level of weight-bearing activity. Again, this shows that it is never too late to start. If you didn't like dealing with ulcers the fist-time around, then you should definitely work to carefully incorporate exercise into your daily routine. The benefits on your overall ability to manage your diabetes coupled with the evidence for avoiding neuropathy and ulcerations should be motivation enough.

If that's not enough motivation for you, listen to this! More and more research has pointed to the subtle cognitive problems that occur in people with diabetes. Now you have to remember that the brain relies almost completely on glucose as its energy source. Further, there is evidence that insulin affects brain function, therefore in cases of insulin resistance when the body starts to produce more insulin to try to get glucose into muscle, fat and liver cells for use or storage, it also is pumping out more insulin that is affecting brain function.

Think about how you feel when you're really hungry, or have just eaten an enormous meal. When you're really hungry you may tend to get a tad bit grouchy and unpleasant to be around. Many folks are very susceptible to changes in, let's say their demeanor when they have low blood sugar. But remember the other side of the coin, when you're totally stuffed, for example after Thanksgiving dinner. In this instance, you may have an experience where you get groggy, start floating in and out of conversations while watching football, and eventually doze off on the couch. These mood states are partially due to wide swings in insulin (and blood sugar), so regulation of this hormone is not something you want to lose complete control over. Exercise can help you keep that control.

Regular exercise also increases our reserve if we need to be sedentary for a few days due to, for example, a hospital stay. A recent study looked at what happened to blood sugar control after three days of bed rest in both exercisers and non-exercisers. After the bed rest period, exercisers maintained tighter control over their blood sugar following a meal. Whereas non-exercisers lost some control due to the bed rest period. This may be a result of the muscles ability to effectively switch the type of fuel it can use even at rest. Since exercisers have built up more muscle they have greater flexibility in fuel choice and have greater reserve for those times when they are unable to exercise regularly.

The ability of exercise to increase sensitivity to insulin also affects people who don't yet have full-blown diabetes (often called pre-diabetes). In this condition, there is a borderline dysregulation of the body's response to insulin, but it hasn't reached the level of full-blown diabetes. Subtle effects on cognition and emotion can occur for these people as well and exercise helps to prevent or correct these lapses.

Parkinson's Disease

Parkinson's disease is a neurodegenerative disorder where dopamine (a neurotransmitter) producing neurons die within a specific region in the brain. The neurons that die are critical for the control of muscular action, which is why individuals with Parkinson's disease experience tremors and other difficulties with movement.

Studies show that a combination of strength (weight) and balance training improves strength and balance in individuals with Parkinson's disease. Further, the effects of strength training persisted after 4-weeks with no training. In fact, there was only a very slight decrease in muscle strength and balance. This is important in the light of the discussion we had above about detraining/atrophy. So even if you miss a couple of weeks of working out, the reserve you built up will carry you through for a little while. Also, having these lasting biological adaptations will make it much easier to make up for lost time once you can get back into your routine.

Very promising news has also come from a study looking at whether exercise or physical activity influences an individual's risk for developing Parkinson's disease. Although this study did not show a strong effect, it suggested positive results are possible. As we talk about these responses to exercise, we have to remember that lifestyle modification affects numerous processes. For example, Parkinson's disease may be a secondary cause for osteoporosis, also known as weak/brittle bones. This is a big problem for people with Parkinson's since they have increased risk for falling. And what happens when people with brittle bones fall? They break bones. Each year in the United States 200,000 people over the age of 65 fall and fracture their hip. Only 16.7% of patients in this age group that sustain hip-fractures regain their full functional ability.

What do hip fractures have to do with exercise and the brain? Well, one of the biological adaptations to exercise is increased density and strength of bones! So for people with Parkinson's disease you get (at least) a quadruple benefit of incorporating weight training into your weekly routine. First, you have the improved signaling from brain to muscle, resulting in more efficient contractions, better coordination, and improved balance. Second, you have improved muscle strength, which will allow you to function better on a day-to-day basis. Third, your bone density, and therefore strength, will increase resulting in lowered risk of fracturing a bone if you do fall. Fourth, you have the improvements in mood and cognition that we have been discussing.

Moving On

We've discussed the importance of physical activity for optimizing our brain-body relationship. We've also explored the value of exercise for people with diseases like Parkinson's and Diabetes. How can you possibly remember all this information? Maybe exercise can help, let's find out what it can do for your memory.

CHAPTER 9

EXERCISING YOUR INTELLECT
Activating Your Cognitive Function

"Oh Lisa, you and your stories. Bart is a vampire. Beer kills brain cells. Now let's go back to that building-thingy, where our beds and TV....is."

- Homer Simpson (Duff Beer aficionado)

It is official, exercise improves intelligence! Well, well, well how the tables have turned. The meek may have inherited the earth, but brawny, and apparently, super-thinking athletes are poised to steal it back in an overtime sudden-death (none of that golden-goal garbage), octagon-of-pain, cage-match!

So what's to become of us now that all those dumb-jocks have the intellectual upper hand? We have already conceded a 48-inch vertical jump to Michael Jordan, the ability to run 40 meters at 1/4 the maximal speed of a cheetah, while dodging 350 pound lineman to Jerry Rice, the ability to carry a small European car 25 meters at a good clip to Magnus Ver Magnusson (aka World's Strongest Man), the pinpoint accurate and physics-defying, ball-bending skills to David Beckham, and a record-setting 8 gold medals in a single Olympics to Michael Phelps. Now these athletic superstars are looking to take the brains with their brawn. Greedy jocks! This will completely change the stereotype. Why can't they just be happy with their brawny glory and leave the brains to the rest of us? Then again, maybe all this worry is a bit premature.

Stupid Like A Fox! A Sedentary Fox.

"Stupid like a fox" is one of many great quotes from the Homer J. Simpson personal library. It's also appropriate, given Homer's level of physical fitness and cognitive capacity, he can serve as the bench-mark of what we don't want to be, no matter how entertaining.

It is becoming very clear that exercise has the ability to improve mental function, particularly in older adults. In addition, there is ample evidence supporting improved test scores and academic performance in children that engage in physical activity. As the research on the topic continues, more evidence is piling up to indicate that older individuals with slight to moderate cognitive impairment reap benefits from increasing their physical activity or by starting to exercise. We don't really know why exercise or physical activity improves cognition. Is it because people decrease their activity as they age, and this makes them more vulnerable to Alzheimer's disease through changes in the way that blood vessels supply the brain with nutrients? Is it that exercise stimulates parts of

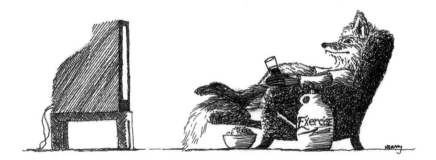

"Although not typically linked with stupidity, this fox appears to be substantially withdrawing from his BrainFit reserves. Maybe he's watching a jazzercise video and getting motivated to make a deposit back into his account."

the brain, or causes changes in our neurochemistry that indirectly keeps our brains active? Does exercise increase our protection against environmental threats like free radicals as discussed in chapter 2? It's probably a combination of all of these things. With these questions fresh in our heads, let's talk about some of the changes that occur with exercise, and how they influence our ability to learn and remember.

Exercise, Fertilizer For The Brain

Plasticity is the ability to change, and is a remarkable property of the brain, given its complexity. It is also a crucial skill of the brain, which underlies the brain's capacity to change and respond to the challenges that we are presented with. It is a vital component allowing us to continue to learn and remember as we age. Plasticity is an incredible and dynamic process that is essential to our survival. We'll revisit plasticity in the context of mental workouts in chapter 13. In this chapter we discuss its role in mediating some benefits of exercise.

Like repaving a road, or building a new one, plasticity in the brain requires resources and energy. It appears that one way this process becomes more efficient is by, again, using it or losing it and there's a trick to it. Once you've done something a few times, you get the hang of it. It becomes easier and takes less focus and effort. This is the result of plasticity in your brain. The trick is that to maintain our brain's capacity for plasticity we need to give it variety. The brain is very good at adapting to challenges and then streamlining the process so that we become efficient at it.

Take typing for example. If you took a formal typing class, you probably remember those days of: fff (space) fff (space) ff (space) ff (space) f (space) f (space), and so on until you learned the location of letters on the keyboard. If you're a heavy user of the keyboard you may recall the first few weeks of trying to type. You'd get going a bit, have to look down to check for a letter or two, but for the most part you could watch the screen as you type, or for us pre-computer typers, the paper (hopefully none of you readers remember the stone and chisel days). It took a lot of focus, coordination, and even self-restraint to keep from looking down at the keys. And then came that magical day where you slipped in your "typing-zone" and blasted out a paragraph with almost uninterrupted clacking as your fingers danced across the keyboard never needing to look down to help them find their targets. Now, if you've been at it for awhile, you're probably much faster at typing than you are at writing with the old pen-and-pad (we hope none of you remember the quill and parchment days). The point being that it took a lot of effort, concentration and tenacity when you first started, but now you don't even think about where the keys are on the keyboard, you just think of the word and let your fingers do the walking.

So what happened? Why the change and why is it that this skill has become essentially unconscious, almost reflexive? Plasticity. This is just one example of how your brain shifts around resources and focus onto a new task. It takes sufficient time and practice to lay-down the new roadwork of connections between brain cells allowing you to efficiently, and almost unconsciously, perform a skill. But now that you're very good at typing you need a new challenge for your brain. It's time to climb the next mountain.

Growth Factors

So you've probably guessed that there is more than magic to this process and that there has to be a fair amount going on behind the scenes of your mind. You're right. Some of the big players in this process are that class of proteins we've talked about before. You guessed it. Growth factors return to the scene to help us out again, the fertilizer for the brain.

We discussed in the last chapter how this class of proteins provide the conditions best suited for growing new connections between brain cells. We've mentioned, a few times, that BDNF increases by exercise. In addition, several other growth factor families increase with exercise (families in the biochemistry world are usually considered as a group of chemicals that have similar structure and do similar types of things in the body). The previously mentioned IGF-1 and VEGF are also involved in learning, memory, and mood regulation. You'll remember that these are also increased with exercise. A new one to add to our list is the Fibroblast Growth Factor (FGF) family. These molecules are part of the machinery that help to repave or lay-down new roadways between brain cells. They are an essential component of learning and memory. When they are blocked, with drugs or other research tools, the synaptic plasticity and ability to learn are disrupted.

Birthing New Brain Cells

A very exciting finding in the past 10 years or so is that exercise has the ability to promote the birth of new brain cells. For a long time, scientist believed that after early childhood the brain no longer had the capacity to produce new brain cells. We now know that's not true. Neurogenesis does happen in specific parts of the adult brain. The hippocampus is a brain region where exercise increases the number of brain cells born, and is also an area that plays an important role in learning and memory. We can't say with certainty that this holds true in the brains of humans yet, but it appears to be very likely. In certain diseases, like Alzheimer's disease, brain cells are dying in the hippocampus, so any potential to produce new brain cells is very promising.

Understanding the role of newly born brain cells for learning and memory is a hot topic of research. In addition, this work promises to lead to therapies for spinal cord injury, and diseases like Parkinson's, which involve damaged or degenerating neurons in specific parts of the nervous system that control movement. But the important thing to take away from this section is that for you, why it helps doesn't really matter (unless you are an active researcher in this field). The important thing is that your body has its own wisdom. You supply it with the ingredients it needs to coordinate all those growth factors to do their jobs and it figures out how to do it. Making physical activity a part of your daily routine is one of those ingredients. You have the ability to produce your own brain fertilizer. If you're able to change your routine every couple months to add a little variety, that's even better. This is another truth to the old adage "variety is the spice of life". Our bodies change to meet challenges. Adaptation is a beautiful thing.

We'd like to point out (again) that the earlier these behaviors are implemented the better your odds for avoiding problems in the future. This may be due to the incorporation of good lifestyle behaviors early in life cause them to become part of a person's routine throughout their life. Another possibility is that we start to develop a reserve as we have talked about in previous chapters, a reserve that will carry us through other difficult times. Just as your financial advisor tells you to put something away now for use later, so goes it for exercises effects on your brain.

Exercise As A Stimulant

Coffee. We're both big fans. It tastes good and has that bit of caffeine that helps nudge us on throughout the day. Some have even credited coffee with providing the spark for the industrial revolution. Caffeine is a stimulant that increases alertness, but there are other effects of this chemical as well. One of the problems that many people experience with coffee is that they usually have one more cup than they need. Sometimes this isn't a problem, but there's always the chance that they will get a little too wound up or develop that "sick buzz" that many of us are familiar with. One of the things many people start to notice as they begin to reprioritizing towards healthy lifestyle is that after they exercise, they feel more awake and alert. In addition, there is less of a chance that we'll experience the 'crash' that occurs with artificial stimulants like caffeine.

The stimulant properties of exercise can also have a down-side. If you exercise within a few hours of your usual bedtime, you'll likely have a hard time falling asleep. However, depending on your schedule, that may be the only option. Trying to make the time for exercise, especially later in the day can seem like an inconvenience, particularly if you're used to burning the candle at both ends. But really how much time does it take, at the most you're dedicating between 7 and 16 hours a week to exercise (if you exercise 30-60 minutes a day and include stretching and changing). And, as time goes on you'll start to realize it is actually very beneficial. By getting into the groove of working out, and then accepting that you need to go to bed when you become tired (instead of drinking coffee to stay up), odds are that your quality of sleep will improve. You'll feel far less groggy when waking up in the morning and you'll dramatically increase your productivity during the day, which will actually allow you to recapture more hours.

Exercise also has the potential to result in increased efficiency when you need to focus on a task. Studies in college students have validated the ability of exercise to increase focus. When college students exercised before studying or before taking a test they showed improvements in test performance. In a lot of ways exercising helped people efficiently burn off excess energy that keeps them up, allowing them to increase their focus and efficiency when working. So some important questions are: How does this happen? And, when is a good time to exercise? We'll talk more about this soon.

Think Of The Children!

One of the saddest things to have happened in organized education in the last two decades is the elimination of physical education classes from many schools. There are a couple of reasons why this seems like such a bad decision. First, this may be the only time some of these kids are getting any physical activity at all. Second, exercise is proven to improve test scores and overall academic performance in children across all subjects. Many studies show positive effects of physical education class on specific aspects of academic performance, including improvements in perceptual skills, intelligence quotient, achievement, verbal tests, mathematic tests, memory, developmental level and academic readiness. These are certainly within the school systems interests. In fact, kids who take PE class do better in all subjects than kids who spend extra time studying those subjects instead of going to PE. Cutting physical activity out of our school programs makes no senses from any perspective that we can think of. To drive the point even further, there is evidence that the earlier you begin good exercise habits the more benefit you will gain over a lifetime.

Arousal, Emotion, And Memory

Arousal (vigilance) increases the likelihood that we will remember things that we are trying to learn. This is an obvious point. Being half asleep makes it much more difficult to be aware of what's going on and to learn. Vigilance is a necessary part of life. For animals, vigilance allows them to be aware of their surroundings so they can avoid predators and other dangers while being aware of rewarding things like food and mates. It should also be no surprise that exercise increases arousal. Therefore, one way for exercise to improve learning is through this very simple response.

Another interesting component of how well we learn is the type of emotional value that we associate with the memory. We discuss this more in chapter 13 in the context of mental activity and learning. Memories that have relatively neutral emotional value tend to be less vivid and less accurately recalled compared to those memories that have strong (positive or negative) emotional value associated with them. Since exercise improves mood and emotional state, this will compliment its effects on learning and memory.

Timing Is Everything

Although most of this chapter has dealt with the effects of long-term exercise habits, some of the short-term biological responses to exercise can improve learning and memory. Even a single session of exercise has the ability to influence an individuals' ability to learn and remember new things. The catch is you have to have the timing down.

A recent study showed the importance and potential value of getting your timing down. Researchers looked at the effect of a single session of exercise of different intensities on student's ability to learn and recall words. Volunteers in this study were asked to sit quietly for 15 minutes, walk at a moderate pace for 40 minutes, or sprint two times for three minutes per sprint. Fifteen minutes after finishing one of those intensities of exercise, they learned a pairing between a made up word and a picture (e.g. glump and a picture of a car). Researchers rated their performance on the speed at which they learned the new pairings, and their accuracy at recalling the pairings at one week, and again at eight months later. That's a pretty long time after learning some new words.

Of the three intensities, the sprinting group learned the pairings 20% faster. So after two sprints of less than three minutes each volunteer's speed of learning was 20% faster compared to the other conditions. In addition, students that sprinted showed greater recall of the word-picture pairings 1-week and 8-months after the single sprint session. Let us repeat that, a single session of two sprints! Although not as dramatic, the walking group also performed better than the sedentary group on some measures of learning. So even if you aren't the sprinting type, going for a walk prior to trying to learn something is probably better than not.

If that weren't enough, the researchers also examined levels of hormones in the blood for potential association with peoples' ability to learn in the word-picture paring task. Levels of BDNF, adrenaline and other hormones involved in our stress-response were elevated after sprinting, or in some cases, walking. Further, these hormones were associated with better short-term and long-term learning success. This indicates that some stress hormones involved in enhanced learning are elevated after intense, but brief, exercise, and to a lesser degree after moderate exercise. See, those stress-hormones aren't always bad (no matter what the infomercials that run at 2am would have you believe), you just need to turn the hormones off when you're done with them.

How did this work? We're not sure. It could be related to changes in attention or vigilance, both of which are affected by the stress-hormones. On the other hand, it may be related to changes in growth factor levels like BDNF that provide a more fertile field for plasticity and synaptogenesis. Maybe it's a little bit of both, any way you look at it, many of us could use a 20% boost in learning every now and again.

Another important point to highlight is that this study was specifically looking at the effect of one session of exercise. There are numerous studies indicating that increasing moderate physical activity as a part of one's daily life has positive benefits on memory, learning and cognition. So don't feel like you need to start incorporating interval sprint work into your daily routine to enhance learning. What we thought was particularly cool about the current study was that it provides another option to try to enhance learning. It also starts to address timing issues of when to learn new things after you have exercised, which we believe could be used to maximize your return on investment.

The old cliché "timing is everything" should be looked upon as a tried-and-true adage. Much of our biology works on a daily rhythm. Along with that, our bodies respond to environmental 'pressures' (eating, exercise, temperature, interacting with other people, etc.) with a variety of finely timed behavioral and biological responses. Basically, when our current state of living is interrupted by some environmental (outside) factor, we will respond until those factors are neutralized. We talk about this more in *Neural Nugget #4, Stressing Out*. However, relevant to this discussion, all of this happens within a narrow window of time. What we are saying is that we may be able to take advantage of these 'altered' states to enhance our ability to hone our cognitive skills.

The above study illustrates how we could capitalize on some of that compensatory biology to do a little multitasking. Get some quick exercise in, and while you're recovering teach yourself a new language learn to solve quadratic equations. Maybe this is a bit of a stretch and maybe it won't work for everyone, or for every type of learning, but the possibilities are there.

Who's Holding The Stop Watch?

A key concept that we can take away from this discussion is the potential for timing of exercise to influence learning. There is clear evidence that the other pillars of brain fitness can influence the ability to learn. We discussed blood sugar regulation by nutrition, which is a big factor. We'll also dig deeper into this during our discussion on mental activity and sleep. The acute effects of exercise appear to have the ability to change our perception and biology in ways that enhance the biological processes of learning.

Can we exploit the timing? It's quite likely that different people will have optimal timing for the interaction between exercise and learning and mood regulation. With the advances in science allowing us to understand more and more about how our genes interact and respond to the environment the ability to screen and deliver personalized timed programs to enhance learning and mood may not be too far off. We will keep our eyes on this exciting area of research for you. Because our understanding of timing and the other fields we cover, continue to change, check the resources section at the end of this book to learn how we can keep you up to date.

Can We Get Too Much Exercise?

Of course, we can get too much of a good thing, which in this case is exercise. It may not be a problem for the majority of us, but we do need to be aware of levels of activity. We should keep in mind the potential for 'unwanted' side effects of exhaustive exercise. Decreases in cognitive function (verbal, as well as immediate and delayed memory) after exercising to exhaustion on a treadmill have been reported, while motor, visual and reaction time were spared. Now, most of us will not exercise to exhaustion (hopefully), however we should really monitor performance in anyone who is trying to optimize their efforts. Actually, this is an important consideration when monitoring people in general. There are direct implications for athletes who will need to undergo neuropsychological testing after a concussion in a sporting event, or for anyone who may be at risk for cognitive problems, from either injury or genetic predisposition.

Often times the people who recognize decreases in performance or function are loved ones and friends, who are really the best at identifying potential problems. The difficulty with relying on the healthcare system to catch problems, is that typically people are tested and compared to some average performance chart. If you test at or above average, a problem won't be suspected by your physician who only sees you once a year and doesn't know you that well. But what if you typically would test at the high end? A drop to just above average might be a sign of a serious problem that would likely go unnoticed. Testing the same individual over time would provide a record of their performance against themselves and may be a more sensitive approach for detecting the early stages of disease than comparing their performance to the statistical average of a group of individuals.

Aging And Alzheimer's

There is clearly a benefit to increasing physical activity early in life, but it's never too late to start. As we age there is a normal impairment in function, but there are two things we need to remember. First, that major impairment seen in neurodegenerative diseases like Alzheimer's is not normal aging. Second, we can reduce the rate and severity of age-related cognitive decline by implementing the four cornerstones of brain fitness.

Many changes occur in our bodies and brains as we age. In the brain, grey-matter loss is associated with normal aging. Loss specifically occurs in several parts of the cortex, involved in memory, planning and several other functions that tend to suffer during aging. However, people with higher aerobic fitness show decreased grey-matter loss, suggesting you can do something about it. Increasing physical activity has also been shown to improve reaction time and executive function in older individuals; and older individuals who are more physically fit have functional performance and brain activation patterns similar to those of younger people. We'll get into other ways of slowing down brain aging in chapters 10-13, as well.

Alzheimer's

The effects of Alzheimer's disease are devastating for those affected by the disease and the people in their lives. However, there is evidence that increasing physical activity can decrease the risk for Alzheimer's disease. More intriguingly, it appears that people who remain physically active during their lives retain their mental capacity even though their brains (upon post-mortem examination) show the pathological signs of Alzheimer's disease. The benefits of physical activity seen in normally aging adults are also evident in people with Alzheimer's disease. In addition, engaging in physical activity during the early stages of Alzheimer's disease has the ability to slow the progression of functional loss.

Active Strategies To Improve Cognitive Performance

The first strategy to improve cognitive performance is to engage in specific times dedicated to exercise. This will increase your overall levels of physical activity. You might ask, why not just increase your physical activity levels? If you can, great! But a lot of times it's difficult to increase your level of physical activity without dedicated exercise. Why? The main reason is time, time, time! For many people there isn't enough of it.

Now, if you do have the time, or you are able to incorporate general physical activity into your life and maintain this behavior, we highly recommend it. In fact, this is the optimal way to start out. There are several reasons for this. First and foremost, figuring out how to incorporate more physical activity into your daily routine will add variety. Even if you only like walking, think of the variety you can implement. You can use different duration, pace, frequency, terrain, time of day, you name it you can try it. Variety coupled with progressive resistance, and balanced with rest, is the key to better performance. This line of thinking can be applied to many aspects of your life. Second, is that physical activity is more amenable to multitasking. Now you could jog into work if it is a reasonable distance, but you'd probably be pretty sweaty depending on the time of year and unless you have a shower and changing facility on-site you may meet some resistance from your co-workers. Walking that distance may take a little longer, but it knocks out the commute and reduces the likelihood that you'll need a shower once you arrive. Even once you have arrived try to sneak in a little more activity. How? Well, instead of sending an email to a co-worker two cubicles over, stand up, walk over and have a conversation with them. Additionally these types of approaches tend to be cheap, which is always an added benefit.

Makin' It More Difficult

I'm betting you have heard the advice about increasing physical activity by not taking advantage of many common technological amenities available in our environment. Elevators, escalators, primo parking spots, the clapper, etc. should be shunned. These changes are a great place to start, especially if you're one of those people who drive their car down to the end of the driveway to get the mail out of the mailbox. One of the most substantial changes to occur over the past 50 to 100 years is the way we interact with our environment on a daily basis.

Back in the good 'ole days, as you may have heard, most people commuted by walking barefoot, uphill both ways in 3 feet of snow. Now aside from the geographical problem of a continual uphill commute implied in this story (requiring a topographical landscape akin to M.C. Escher's *Relativity*), there were probably at least a couple of snow-free weeks during the year. In reality, however, there is a good deal of truth to these stories. In chapter 6 we mentioned a very interesting study published by Brownson and colleagues in 2005. To remind you, this study analyzed databases reporting lifestyle information from the 1950's through the year 2000, including a variety of measures estimating physical activity. It highlights some of the scary changes we have witnessed and experienced; including a 71% drop in the number of people commuting to work on foot.

This is due to several factors such as suburbanization, but that doesn't stand alone. Yes, many of us live farther away from work but we have also become lazy. We drive our personal vehicles right up to the door, instead of taking busses or trains and walking from the station. We drive to lunch, even if its within walking distance. Some even drive to get their mail! We drive everywhere. If you haven't seen the movie *LA Story*, it's highly worth checking out since it speaks to this issue in a very humorous way.

In addition, the Brownson study found a dramatic reduction in the number of people with occupations requiring relatively high levels of physical activity, further contributing to our declining energy expenditures. We won't even terrify you with the increase in hours of television watched per day. So this study suggests that compared to 1950 we're not physically active on our way to or from work. We're not physically active while we're at work and we're probably not all that physically active once we get home from work if we're sitting in front of the idiot box. These factors have helped lead us to where we are now, trying to squeeze in chunks of time completely dedicated to exercise with the goal of contributing to our overall physical activity levels.

One caveat to increasing your activity by making things a little more difficult is that once you've done it for awhile your body will adapt and you won't continue to obtain physiological benefits. You'll likely maintain what you've gained, but you won't make substantial improvements. Once you reach this point, where you'll likely not feel much physical challenge, you'd do well to pick things up a bit or change up your routine so you can continue to improve until you reach whatever physical fitness goal you may have.

Multitasking Technology

Let's return to the issue of time for a minute. In talking with friends and colleagues about the time investment required to complete a workout, a similar story continues to pop-up. For example, if you need to go to a gym to get your walk or jog on, because it is five degrees Fahrenheit outside (-23 degrees Fahrenheit with wind-chill), you realize it is a multi-step ordeal. Here is the scenario for most people: First, you need to change into workout clothes either before you leave the house or once you're at the gym. Second, you need to drive there, park, get into the building and stow your triple fat goose-down-arctic-snorkel-coat, because the frozen spinach and chicken cutlets in your freezer are in a warmer environment than the one you just drove through. Third, if you are one of those unlucky souls that has to frequent the gym during peak hours (6-8am, 12-1pm, or 5-7pm) due to your work schedule, your odds of walking in and onto your equipment of choice are slightly better than winning the multi-state power-ball jackpot. Now, once you've finished you have to commute to your next destination (work, home, ice-fishing hut, wherever). It's no wonder that more folks aren't beating down the doors to sign up for this. It takes approximately 1.5 hours to complete 30 to 45 minutes of actual exercise. Please understand, this is time well spent. But what if we could maximize our efficiency? There is another way.

Do The Work Yourself

There are a variety of machines and gadgets that are coming to the market that will give us the opportunity to increase our physical activity. Things like computer workstations built around treadmills, a motorized tire that can be placed on any standard bicycle (just the tire has a motor in it), even knee braces that turn our movements into energy that can be used to power our cell phones and iPods. Some of these are available now, and some are coming on-line in the near future. Be creative, there are plenty of options out there. All of these provide an opportunity to turn times when you would normally be sedentary into times of moderate activity.

Imagine, standing on a treadmill moving at 0.5 m.p.h. while you're working on your computer (we sure could have used that writing this book). Imagine having a bicycle that you can flip the small motor on for longer or more difficult commutes and then flip it off to do a little work yourself. We're not talking about big clunky mopeds here, but sleek small and light road bikes. People are already incorporating these technologies into their lives to return physical activity to modern-day schedules, and more technologies are coming. It's sort of ironic really. We need technology to get us out of a mess that technology put us into in the first place.

Exercising Spatial Awareness And Balance

A final topic we want to discuss in this chapter surrounds your brain's spatial awareness of your body. To demonstrate this property, close your eyes and move one of your hands to shoulder level. Then, without looking, do you have an idea of where your hand is? This non-visual awareness of our body (limbs, etc.) in space is referred to as proprioception. Think about how useful this is on a daily basis. You're cutting up that churoso for your Mexican breakfast omelet with your brand new 9-inch Henkles chef knife while you're talking with your brother-in-law. You could also substitute a smoked pork-shoulder if a barbeque analogy would hold your attention better. Wouldn't it be great to not cut the tips of your fingers off? With proprioceptive processes, we have an awareness (not always conscious) of where our body is in space. Where our hands are when we're catching a ball, where our feet are when we're walking, etc. Given that the risk of falling dramatically increases as we age and is a serious cause of injury in older adults, this skill would be great to maintain.

A potential way to improve this sense is by practicing tasks that improve coordination, prediction, and timing. Let's use juggling as an example. Now you may not want to start off juggling machete's or chainsaws, which could result in disfigurement or dismemberment. But juggling a few bean-bags or tennis balls requires attention, prediction and the coordination of multiple limbs. This helps keep brain circuits that control proprioception active and challenged, to maintain coordination and control.

Maintaining vestibular function, or balance, is also incredibly important, especially as we age. Not only in our everyday lives, but for things like walking and not falling. The American College of Sports Medicine has incorporated balance training into its suggested exercise regimen for anyone over the age of 65. This is an essential component for aging peoples' physical activity routines, but balance training is really a great endeavor for people of all ages. In fact, several sports and beneficial exercises are based on the premise of disrupting or maintaining balance. Tai Chi and Yoga are great examples. They challenge you to hold poses to enhance your strength and balance and they differ greatly from 'traditional' forms of exercise, like walking, running, lifting weights, or swimming. So proprioception and vestibular function are two great terms to add to your crossword puzzle arsenal, and to your daily routine to maintain strength, coordination and balance throughout life.

Moving On

In this section, we explored the benefits that our brains receive from exercising our bodies. Hopefully, we've shown you the benefits of physical activity and exercise on many aspects of cognitive function. Realize that the earlier you start the more you'll get out of it, but it's never too late to begin. Also, there are many options, and variety is of the utmost importance. So engage, explore, and get physically active for your minds' sake.

In the next section of the book, we'll delve into how mental workouts boost your total EPIC performance.

TALLYING THE SCORE FOR EXERCISE:
BRAIN FITNESS – 1, BRAIN DECLINE – 0

Hopefully this section has provided you with some background on the importance of incorporating physical activity as part of your daily routine. Remember, exercise can help a lot of things, but you have to actually do it! It must become a prioritized part of your life.

Key Concepts:

- Exercise has profoundly positive effects on your brain and body.
- The sooner you start the better, but it's never too late. Studies in older individuals report substantial benefits of exercise for brain function.
- Exercise improves moods in people with and without mood disorders.
- Exercise improves learning, memory and cognition in people of all ages.
- Exercise reduces stress.
- Our environment has changed dramatically in the past few decades, requiring less daily activity. This has created a new set of challenges and problems that you need to be aware of so you can effectively address them.
- We have an inherent drive to maintain energy stores in case of famine (FAT PADS). You can directly reduce your PADS by supplementing your activity levels.
- These changes may be difficult at first, but stick with it. Physical activity will become easier with time. After a few months you'll wonder how you ever did without it.

Key Action Points:

- Check with your physician to make sure you are healthy enough to start exercising particularly if you are making a major change in your routine or have not been active for a long time.
- Start slow and listen to your body. No one knows your body better than you do.
- Figure out what physical activities you like to do and make them a priority. Don't cheat yourself! These are deposits into your Brain-Fitness reserve account.
- Balance, variety, and creativity are key.
- Change your routine once it becomes easy.
- Remember that rest is important. Insufficient rest and recovery can lead to injury which may require extended periods of recovery. Extended recovery will disrupt your ability to stay active.
- Find a partner or a group to exercise with, to make yourself accountable for workouts and help you succeed during difficult times.
- Whenever possible make your exercise social, and your physical activity part of other daily duties. Multitask for efficiency, but don't devalue physical activity or exercise.

The Third Cornerstone

Mental Activity

CHAPTER 10

MIND GAMES

Introduction To Mentally Activating Your Brain Fitness

"Cultivation to the mind is as necessary as food is to the body".
- Marcus Tillius Cicero, circa 500 B.C. (philosopher)

Mental activity means many things. It includes anything from tying your shoes and navigating your way across your living room, to solving mathematical equations modeling the expansion of the universe. Mental activity can also include positive thinking, visualization or just sitting quietly in reflection. You can't help but use your mind every day. You use it when you are awake or asleep; when you are at home or at work; when you are angry and when you are happy. The thing to understand is that using your mind, changes the physical structure of your brain. Thoughts are things. They are electro-chemical pulses that by their very existence modify the brain circuits through which they move. Your mind is constantly working and modifying itself and the brain that contains it. However, not all changes are for the better. To improve your mind, you need to do more than just use it. You need to challenge it.

You may have heard that we only use 10 to 20 percent of our brain. This is a myth. There is no untapped compartment in their waiting to be discovered through some magical experience. We use our entire brain. However, there is some truth to that statement in a couple of different ways. First, you don't use your entire brain all of the time. If you did, you would be utterly confused. Your brain, in this sense, is like an orchestra. If all the strings, brasses and percussions were going full tilt all the time, it would sound horrible. There would be no detectable melody or rhythm. Your brain is similar in that the different parts of your brain need to come on- and off-line at coordinated times to do all the things you need to do. So, in this sense, you are only using some smaller percentage of your brain at any given time. Second, and related to this, you can improve the efficiency and skill that you use to coordinate all of the parts of your brain. You could give all of the same instruments to your middle-school orchestra and to the New York Philharmonic. Even though they would have identical tools, which one would sound better? From this perspective there's no question that we can all improve the way we use the brain tools that we have.

Your mind is like a muscle in its ability to gain or lose strength. The more you nurture it, exercise it and give it the appropriate rest and recovery time, the stronger it can become. However, it will only get stronger at the skills that you work on. When you lift weights with your arms, the muscle fibers in your arms get stronger; but the muscles in your legs don't benefit. If you want to increase the strength of your leg muscles, you must work them out directly.

Similarly, you have circuits in your brain, made up of neurons connected to each other. Different circuits control different things. Some control cognitive skills, like memory, vocabulary, logic, decision-making and creativity. Other circuits control positive and negative emotions. Some circuits control movement, like balance, coordination and agility. And still others control physiological functions like heart rate, breathing rate, digestion and immune response. To strengthen any of these circuits you have to engage in activities that use those circuits. Also, like a muscle, if you stop using *or misuse* circuits, they can weaken and become less efficient and effective.

Road Maps Of The Mind

Think of brain circuits as a system of roads in your mind. The roads connect different parts of the brain that need to talk to each other in order to accomplish specific tasks. Just like roads in our society change over time, our brain circuits change throughout our lives. Several hundred years ago, most of the roads in our society were dirt trails. The roads that proved useful drew heavy traffic and the dirt trails widened and 'strengthened'. Roads not used over-grew and disappeared. As our society 'aged' and our technological abilities progressed, we put more demand on our roads. The automobile became commonplace and the useful roads were improved and paved. Some of them became highways and freeways. The more traffic they received, the more stable and faster the roads became. Others went unused, and society left them to decay. Importantly, even roads that were once popular and maintained fell into disrepair and degeneration if they went unused for long periods.

Route 66 is part of American lore. It was the major 'circuit' connecting Chicago to Los Angeles and all the Midwest hubs in between. However, as society progressed and the national highway system improved, we no longer needed this circuit. It became irrelevant and unused and society left many parts of the highway to degenerate. Some sections remain intact today, for historical purposes. Other sections survive as pieces of the newer highway system, but for the most part the route has been dismantled. Not only that, many communities that thrived on route 66 became ghost towns as traffic diverted to more efficient highway systems.

Brain circuits are similar, as you develop from young childhood to adulthood. Your brain will stabilize and 'ramp-up' the circuits that prove useful. As you age, your brain will also allow circuits that go unused to degenerate, or even actively dismantle them. As we've discussed previously your brain uses about 20% of your body's energy and, in terms of space and energy, it is very costly to continue to maintain brain circuits that are not used. So your brain sees them as unnecessary and diverts that energy to circuits that are used. The older we get, the more our brain circuits tend to degenerate, and the less we make the necessary road improvements. One way to counter this process, however, is to drive traffic down those brain circuits with an active mind, so you continue to 'vote' for their maintenance and improvement.

To make a final point, continuing with the road analogy, we all have different road maps. The major freeways and highways in our brains are the same for all of us. These are genetically programmed features of the human brain. We all have the same major brain parts and major circuitry connecting those parts. However, the small circuits (the side roads) are different in all of us. These circuits are by design, highly flexible and easily remodeled. We need to have flexibility in our brain circuits so that we can adapt to our environment. If everything were 'hard-wired' we would have a difficult time dealing with any kind of change.

Bridging The Gap

One way to increase the strength of a brain circuit is to make more synapses, which are small gaps that connect neurons in a circuit. For simplicity, think of a brain signal moving through a circuit as a baton, passed from runner to runner. The baton (brain signal) starts with one runner (neuron), who carries it for some distance and then passes it to the next runner (next neuron). The points at which the neurons pass the baton are the synapses.

When an electrical signal moves from one end of the neuron to the other, the neuron passing the signal releases a chemical message into the synapse. These chemicals cross the synaptic gap to activate specific receivers (called receptors) on the next neuron. Once received, the signal turns back into an electrical impulse and travels down that neuron to the next synapse in the circuit. So the process goes from electrical impulse moving down a neuron (like a wire), to a chemical pulse across the synaptic gap (like passing a baton), back to an electrical pulse down the next neuron, and so on. This process continues from electrical to chemical to electrical to chemical, until the baton (brain signal) reaches its destination. This is why we call the brain an electro-chemical organ.

Now here's the part that you can work on. Not all synapses are equally effective. Some are very weak, meaning they don't always release enough chemicals (called neurotransmitters) into the synapse. When this occurs, they fail to activate the next neuron and the signal dies. This is sort of like placing a cell phone call in an area where you don't have many bars. The weaker the signal, the more you are likely to drop the call; the stronger the signal, the more likely you are to have a clear, uninterrupted conversation. A strong synapse will allow an uninterrupted signal as well.

An active mind strengthens connections between neurons in a couple of ways. First, using a brain circuit regularly can cause a neuron to release more neurotransmitter into the synapse. This increases the chance the next neuron will receive the signal, activate, and carry the message forward.

Essentially, the synapse gets stronger and more effective. Second, regular use of a brain circuit can cause two connected neurons to make more synapses through which they can talk to

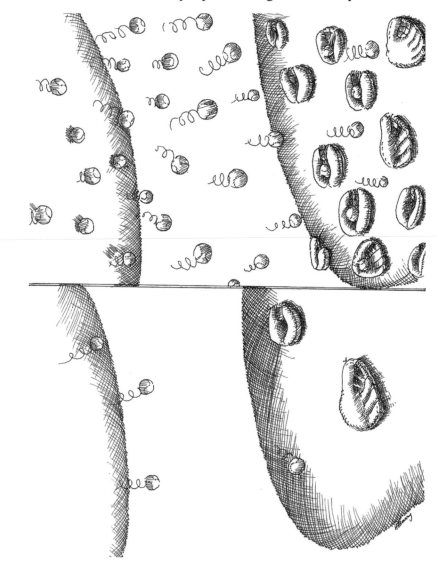

"A strong synapse has more 'transmitters' and 'receivers' to get a message across the gap. Mental activities can help strengthen the synapses in the brain."

each other (a process called synaptogenesis, literally meaning 'synapse creation'). Think of this as multiple bridges over a river to increase the connectivity between the two sides. If one bridge fails or undergoes repairs, others can pick up the traffic. Third, neurons can make synapses with other neurons they weren't originally talking to and recruit more brain cells into the circuit. Again, all of these increase the odds that the signal will not get dropped. Importantly, these strategies also increase the stability of the brain circuit, making it less likely to degenerate or get dismantled as you age.

Your brain is constantly employing all of these tactics, all of the time. It is continually testing out new connections to see how useful they are. It then stabilizes the ones that work and dismantles the ones that don't. In fact, there is a saying in neuroscience that "neurons that fire together, wire together". Meaning, if a bunch of brain cells are always responding to the same thing (firing together), they will tend to form a team to do a better job (wire together).

Admittedly, we've presented the above discussion in an oversimplified form. Actual circuits in the brain aren't formed by one neuron talking to another, but by thousands. You have approximately 100 billion neurons in your brain and each has an average of about 10,000 connections, or synapses. This means that a single neuron can actually pass thousands of 'batons' to thousands of other neurons at the same time. Neurons talk to each other in a very complex web, which is constantly undergoing restructuring to find the best way to accomplish the tasks that you ask it to perform.

This is what neuroscientists refer to as 'plasticity', which is the flexibility to change and adapt to whatever it is asked to do. This is why the human brain has been able to function in environments as different as cave man times to modern technology, without a change in design. Our brains are incredibly flexible in their ability to learn and excel in our environment.

Some scientists believe that the highly flexible nature of the human brain, which allows us to be such an intelligent species, is also the reason why we seem more susceptible to Alzheimer's disease and dementia as we age. If you think about this, it makes sense. It's like comparing a brick to silly putty. A brick is very stable, but won't fit into a crack that you'd like to fill. In contrast, silly putty is very plastic, but if you placed some weight on it, it would squish. The point being, you can't have high stability and high flexibility at the same time. It's a trade-off. Because of this instability, as we age these flexible circuits are more likely to destabilize and breakdown. However, we don't have to stand by and watch this happen. We can take advantage of this flexibility as we age to help keep our minds sharp. We can continue to do things that challenge and maintain brain circuit strength and stability, which is what this book is all about.

A Star Is Born (or at least a neuron shaped like one)

Beyond making new connections and rewiring the neurons that you have, your brain is also continually making new neurons, a process called 'neurogenesis' (literally meaning 'neuron creation'). Until recently, this was a very controversial area of neuroscience and still remains somewhat debated. A couple of decades ago scientific dogma was that you did not make new neurons after early childhood. You get what you get and you don't get no more. So if you killed off a few thousand neurons in a college drinking binge, too bad.

However, we now know that's not really true. Evidence began to emerge that neurogenesis (the birth of new neurons) happens in specific parts of the brain in adults. Still, this topic remained highly controversial and required scientists to revisit beliefs that we had held firm for a long time. Today, the data are rather overwhelming that neurogenesis occurs on a regular basis throughout adulthood, at least in some parts of the brain, but many details are yet to be unveiled.

Two areas of the brain that clearly birth new brain cells on a regular basis are the hippocampus (involved in learning and memory) and the olfactory system (involved in the sense of smell). Outside of these regions, data are weaker but there is some indication that other parts of the brain perform neurogenesis as well, including the cortex (involved in higher levels of thinking) and the hypothalamus (involved in regulating much of the rest of the body).

Neurogenesis is currently a hot topic of research and we are really only beginning to understand how it works. Hopes are that we can use this property of the brain to help treat neurodegenerative diseases, like Alzheimer's, Parkinson's and multiple sclerosis, as well as spinal cord and traumatic brain injuries. The trick, whether treating disease or improving normal everyday brain function, is to get the new neurons to incorporate into the brain circuits that will do you the most good. It's great to recruit all these new 'players', but you want to get them to join the right 'team' to be effective.

As discussed in Section II on physical activity, exercise is key factor that regulates the rate of neurogenesis. Regular physical activity can boost the number of new neurons born, at least in the hippocampus. Mental activity, on the other hand, is likely a key factor on incorporating these newly born neurons into the appropriate brain circuits. Above, we discussed how the brain is constantly testing new synaptic connections. This is especially true for newly born neurons that need to find a home in the appropriate circuit. If new neurons get into an under-used circuit, there is little incentive for them to survive.

However, if they join a growing team that gets regular use and metabolic attention (blood flow and nutrient delivery), they may incorporate themselves and thrive. The hope is, as we learn more about this process we will be able to guide new neurons to the best locations. For now, simply keeping an active mind, as we will discuss throughout this section, is a great start.

Walking The Tightrope

Like anything else in life, improving your neural circuitry through mental activity is about balance. Generally, there are two kinds of mental experiences. First, new experiences help you make new connections. We discussed how synaptogenesis and neurogenesis help neurons link up and talk to each other. Second, repeated experiences help make existing connections stronger and faster. We discussed how existing communication between neurons can improve reliability. Your brain will serve you best when you keep these two types of mental activities in balance.

Life-long learning to constantly engage your mind in new experiences is a big factor in late-life mental health. However, if you don't spend enough time mastering a single topic, you are less likely to establish the strong stable brain circuits discussed above. You don't want to be a jack of all trades, but master of none. Similarly, if you spend all your time ultra-focused on mastering a narrow skill set, you are less likely to build a variety of skills, which can help protect you from dementia as you age. We'll discuss these concepts more in chapter 13. Again, balance is key.

Your brain is heavily invested in balancing the fortification of useful connections while at the same time dismantling inappropriate ones. We have already discussed how you can make new connections and strengthen them. But there is another side to the coin, a Yin to the Yang. Sometimes your brain needs to dismantle connections that aren't working correctly or simply aren't used much. Your brain needs to keep house by cleaning up the mess every now and then. If you kept every experience you ever had at the forefront of your mind you wouldn't be able to focus on anything and life would be very difficult.

Throughout development and into adulthood your brain actively prunes some of the connections in order to keep everything running smoothly. Just like you prune a tree or a bush to keep it growing well, your brain prunes neuronal 'branches' to ensure circuits are kept in good working order. In fact, one theory of schizophrenia is that their brains don't appropriately prune unnecessary connections and their thoughts get all 'tangled up'.

Schizophrenics, contrary to popular belief, don't have multiple personalities. That is a completely different disorder. But schizophrenics have difficulty separating reality from fantasy. They may hear voices, see visions or experience things that aren't real. If you've ever seen the movie, *A Beautiful Mind*, you'll have some insight into what a schizophrenic experiences. This movie did a great job of depicting what it's like for some schizophrenic patients.

Normally, your immune system plays a role in pruning brain circuits to ensure they don't get out of control. Some scientists believe that this process doesn't work correctly in schizophrenic brains. That somehow the immune system is not pruning brain circuits correctly in the schizophrenic brain and this leads to cross-wiring and short-circuits that shouldn't occur. This is still only a theory, but there is a good deal of evidence for altered immune system function in the brains of schizophrenic patients.

The point of this discussion is that balance is a key part of brain fitness. You can always get too much of a good thing. Neurogenesis and synaptogenesis to create new neurons and new connections between neurons are great to maintain a sharp mind. But growth for the sake of growth is the ideology of a cancer cell, and that is never a good thing. Balancing new experiences and life-long learning, with development of expertise and mastery, is a key part of boosting your EPIC performance.

The Social Ties That Bind

We point out the value of a socially supportive network for the other cornerstones throughout this book. Social support helps with adherence to any healthy lifestyle program, whether for improved diet, increased exercise or better sleep habits. Accountability is a key factor for success. However, the role of social support in brain fitness deserves special attention in this section on mental activity. Social support systems in and of themselves have proven beneficial for maintaining physical and mental health in late life.

Engaging in social networks is beneficial for physical and mental health. Strong social networks seem to protect against cardiovascular disease, Alzheimer's disease and depression. The likely explanations for these protective effects include increased mental activities and challenging leisure activities as well as reduced overall stress in socially supported people. The opposite is also true. Social isolation can lead to more rapid cognitive decline and depression.

Importantly, social contact is not sufficient. The social network must be supportive, giving people a sense of control over their interactions. This means that living in a community surrounded by others is not enough. Positive social groups may be faith-based organizations, family, recreational and leisure groups, or a close network of friends. Whereas, institutional environments can sometimes be negative if the patient or resident has no sense of control.

Evidence also suggests that the positive affect of social networks spreads across life, from childhood to old age. Meaning, like nearly everything else that's good for your health, the earlier you get started in positive social networks the better, but it's never too late to start. People, after all, are social animals. Most of us have a desire to be around other people at least some of the time, even though you might feel like people drive you nuts at other times. Still, you need them and they need you for life-long brain health and fitness.

But what if you don't have a strong social network? Today's internet technology places a social network literally at your fingertips. Studies have shown that even internet chat groups provide significant benefit for improving measures of psychological and physical well being. Importantly, the design of many social networking sites keeps the novice internet user in mind and requires very little in the way of learning computer skills (although learning these skills is an added benefit for your brain). In today's environment, there is no reason to be alone. There are one billion people on-line worldwide and hundreds of social networking sites that cater to specific needs, interests and age groups. The resource section at the end of this book can get you started.

Moving On

The remainder of this section focuses on how mental activities relate to cognitive, emotional and physical functions of your brain and body. You can have incredibly healthy and vibrant neurons connected up with thousands of others, but optimizing your EPIC performance comes down to teamwork. Just like building a good sports team, it takes practice to get everyone working together.

Let's find out how to do that.

Neural Nugget #4 – Stressing Out

The Good, Bad And The Ugly Of Stress

We've discussed stress a few times in this book. However, the topic of stress is so important that it warrants some deeper digging in its own neural nugget. Most people think of stress as a bad thing, and often it is. Yet there are many times when stress is good, so we really need to understand the difference. After all, we did not develop an entire 'stress response system' just to hinder our health. Stress has important positive functions as well.

The concept of stress in its current form stemmed from pioneering work of a psychologist named Hans Seyle in the mid 1950's in a paper titled 'What is Stress?' Since this time, psychologists and physiologists have been debating the definition and we're not about to solve that debate here. However, we can put stress into some very broad terms to help you understand why it's not always bad.

Scientists often view stress as the activation of what's called the hypothalamic-pituitary-adrenal (HPA) axis, although this is not always true. We couldn't really consider ourselves neuroscientists if we didn't offer at least a simplified overview of the HPA axis in a discussion about stress so we'll digress for a minute down that path. However, we promise to keep it brief.

Stressors come from many sources, psychological and physical. Regardless, stress culminates with your brain's master hormone regulator, the hypothalamus, releasing a hormone called CRH, which makes its way a short distance to your pituitary gland. Your pituitary obeys the signal from the hypothalamus by releasing another hormone, called ACTH, into the blood stream. ACTH makes its way to your adrenal glands (sitting just on top of your kidneys), which also obey and release adrenaline and cortisol into your blood stream. These two hormones go off to have all sorts of effects, including activating your sympathetic nervous system, which is responsible for your fright, flight or fight response. OK – that's it for the biology.

Whether or not stress is a good thing or a bad thing depends on many factors. First, it depends on the source of the stress. For example, starvation is stressful for your body and is not a healthy endeavor. However, exercise is also stressful for your body but that is certainly not bad for you. Second, it depends on the duration of the stress. Worrying for half a day about your performance on tomorrow morning's driver's test, might get you focused and on your toes. But worrying about the direction your kids have been going down for the last five years is not doing you much good. Third, and probably most importantly, is the amount of control you have to affectively change your stressor. Stressing out on your job is not uncommon for many people today. But in the end, you can work to change your work situation and effectively reduce your stress. Granted, that can be very difficult, but is still within your power and this knowledge helps you stay sane. Conversely, subjecting yourself to the violent behavior of your cellmate, who you're trapped in prison with for the next decade, is completely out of your control, and can be very damaging to your psyche.

Your perception of how much control you have in a situation is also important. You may feel completely helpless, when in fact you are not. Conversely, you may have the strength to control your own thoughts, even in the worst of situations. The book, Man's Search for Meaning, *by Victor*

Frankl, details his refusal to allow his oppressors to control his mind in his battle for survival as a concentration camp prisoner during the Holocaust. It is an incredible account about the power of a focused mind.

Even accounting for these types of factors, some people will respond positively to stress (adaptive) while others will respond negatively (maladaptive) when faced with the same situation. To some degree, your personality type accounts for how you will respond to certain stressors. For example, if you are a Type-A control freak faced with a situation where you are forced to relinquish a little control, you may not handle it too well. You are more likely to have a prolonged activation of a stress response that puts you at increased risk for cardiovascular illness. On the other hand, if you are a calm Type-B person, you may handle minor changes in control much better. Conversely, if you are placed in a situation of injustice, the Type-A person may step up and put a stop to it and end the stress, whereas the Type-B person may back down and let it fester, boosting their odds of developing depression. In one scenario it's better to be Type-A, while in the other scenario, Type-Bs have a health advantage.

In chapter four, we discussed the concept of homeostasis, which is your body's attempt to keep itself in a stable state. You need to keep your temperature at 98.6 degrees, your blood sugar in a tight range, your blood pressure under control, etc. Any perturbations to the system activate some level of a stress response to bring it back under control. It's as if your brain sends out an alarm to tell your body to handle whatever perturbation is the problem. Minor stressors may send out a 'code yellow' whereas major stressors may send out a 'code red', especially if the stress involves a life or death situation. So from this perspective, stress is good. It's a way to get you out of trouble and return to normal.

Problems happen when the stress response gets out of control and stays active for too long. Some have likened it to firefighters pouring water on a fire. You need enough water to put the fire out, but if you continue to dump buckets of water after the flames are extinguished then the situation is made worse by causing unnecessary water damage. Also, if the firemen pour on the water for too long the water pressure will drop and there may not be enough in the system to fight the fire that crops up a block away. Again, it comes back to balance. Just enough stress to deal with the problem but not too much.

Some of this is under your control, either psychologically or physically. Good nutrition and exercise have a big impact on how your body deals with stress physiologically. A good mental attitude and enough sleep impact how you deal with stress psychologically. However, as we discussed in the various chapters, they all relate at some level to both physical and psychological control.

Stress can also be good from another perspective and that is to challenge your system. We talk about challenging your mind in chapter 13 in order to improve it. We talk about challenging your body in chapter 8. Whenever you challenge yourself (which is stressful) you increase your physical or psychological skills a little bit. Someone training for a marathon will not just go run 26.2 miles right off the bat. They slowly increase their distance over months of training, challenging their bodies and increasing their skills. Distances that once were extremely difficult become routine and easy. This type of stress is good.

There are some interesting studies looking at protecting the brain from low oxygen. Typically, a stroke will cause brain damage (sometimes reversible) by cutting off the oxygen supply to a part of the brain for a brief period. However, in animal studies, if researchers subject a rat to small periods of oxygen reduction, but not enough to cause brain damage, their brains will adapt. Now if that animal experiences a stroke that would normally cause brain damage, they will recover without problems. Their brains were 'stressed' in small ways so they could adapt to bigger challenges.

The message here is that if you never expose yourself to stress at all (which may be impossible anyway) then you don't provide yourself with the opportunity to grow. In the words of Batman's butler Alfred: "Why do we fall Master Bruce? So that we can learn to pick ourselves back up." The bottom line is that it's all about a cost-benefit analysis. Stress is good if you can turn it off when the stressor is gone, and you actually emerge stronger. Stress is bad if you can't turn it off or don't remove yourself from the situation that is causing you stress. You will do more damage than good and your fire hoses will eventually run out of water.

CHAPTER 11

CALM YOUR QUALMS
Mental Activity For Emotional Intelligence

"People in good moods are better at creative problem solving"
- Daniel Goleman (author and psychologist)

Using your mind to control your mood and emotional state is both the realm of clinical psychiatry and popular psychology. Part of this chapter will focus on hard data from the clinical world and part will discuss some ideas from popular psychology, including success and personal development. After all, not everything has been tested by science, nor is everything testable. The biggest example of an untestable theory is, of course, the existence of God. This is outside the scientific domain. We will never prove or disprove the existence of God by scientific measures. But that does not mean God cannot exist. Believers must rely on their own faith to guide them.

We make every effort to bring scientific-based approaches into discussions throughout this book. However, we also do not want to omit important topics from discussion just because they lack hard data. Many topics are still worthy of bringing up and putting on the table. Science has not yet pursued many aspects of our world, especially when it comes to the human mind. We have much left to understand. For this reason, science should not discount popular theories as impossible, simply because we don't have the mental capacity, the technology or the knowledge base to understand how they can be possible. In fact, we believe to do so is arrogant.

It wasn't that long ago that we believed the Earth was flat and at the center of the Universe. This was an undisputed fact and anyone who thought differently was a crackpot. Today this seems absurd. Yet Europeans became aware of the new world and the roundness of the earth less than 600 years ago. That's only a blink of an eye on the scale of human history. Even more recently, we burned people at the stake convinced that they were witches, and we felt completely justified and correct to do it. That was only a couple of hundred years ago. These actions seem almost unbelievable by today's knowledge.

In the high tech science world of biotechnology, we are still making discoveries about the nature of life's inner workings. Sometimes discovering entire systems that we had no idea existed even a decade ago. One glaring example was the discovery that the human genome contains only about 20,000 genes. This is about ten times fewer than the number we estimated from some good scientific logic prior to the human genome project. Now we know better. What beliefs do we hold true today that we will expose tomorrow as sheer ignorance? As the famous quote goes, "Your mind is like a parachute, it only works when it is open".

Now, just because we make the argument to keep an open mind does not mean that we suggest you should blindly accept a snake-oil salesman's offerings. We must think critically, especially when science provides evidence against specific theories. We must also think for ourselves and accept what we believe to be true and what our own personal experience best supports. This is not the same as dismissing possibilities due to lack of supporting data. Evidence against, and lack of evidence for, are two completely different things. So when it comes to working on your own mind, if you find value in a certain approach, there is no reason to wait for the data to support it. However, if data emerges to discount your approach, you may want to reconsider the investment of your time, energy and possible finances.

Power Of Positive Thinking

For decades, the personal development industry has been preaching the power that your mind has on your ability to reach your goals, including emotional strength and stability. Even though this lacks hard data-driven support, there is likely something very real to this. The human mind is amazing at creating its own reality. There are volumes of books written on this topic, dealing with everything from simple positive attitudes, to affirmations, to the law of attraction, detailed in the recent blockbuster, *The Secret*.

It's easy to buy into the potential benefits of a positive attitude from a neuroscience perspective. The more time you spend activating brain circuits with a positive outlook, the more stable they become and the easier it is to enter a positive emotional state. Belief in the power of affirmations and the law of attraction, however, requires a little more faith, but some swear by their effectiveness. With affirmations, you are supposed to hold a vision in your mind of exactly what you want your life to look like to increase your odds of achieving it. The more specific, tactile and emotionally charged the vision, the better. The law of attraction states that by using affirmations, your mind will 'attract' opportunities to you to make them come true.

Whether or not this is possible, we don't know. There is certainly no real scientific data to support it. However, as discussed above this is not reason enough to discount the possibility. But there is a *component* of the law of attraction that can be explained through neuroscience terms. Your brain will pay attention to opportunities that come your way if you interpret them as important. By focusing your mind on what you want, your mind will be 'on alert' to look for ways to get you there.

Life confronts you with hundreds of opportunities to act on every day. If you have been using affirmations on a regular basis, you are much more likely to notice opportunities that will lead you to your goal; opportunities that you may have missed or dismissed otherwise. In addition, consistently recognizing those opportunities will likely strengthen your resolve to achieve your goal. Whether or not you can actually attract those opportunities is a completely different question that you must answer for yourself on faith. But you certainly can affect the probability that you will take action on those that do come your way.

Most of us go through much of our life in automatic mode. We have routines that we get into everyday that remove opportunities from our mental horizon. You probably wash yourself in the shower in the same sequence everyday; get dressed in the same order; brush your teeth in the same way; make breakfast in some similar sequence, even if you are eating different things in the morning. This continues throughout the day, probably taking the same route to work; go through the same ritual of settling into your office; and on and on.

This autopilot mode disengages your mind from paying attention to the present. You have done your routine so many times that you have no need to think about what you're doing, it's automatic. By disengaging your mind, you most certainly miss subtle opportunities throughout your day. In a way, this is somewhat necessary. You can't notice or act on everything. You'd be distracted, unfocused and get nothing done. But, at the same time, if you slip too deeply into a routine you will miss opportunities that may help you achieve your goals. Taking some time each day to focus on what you want your life to look like will put your mind on notice, and help you wake up from your routine when appropriate opportunities arise.

Emotional intelligence plays back into this because whenever you associate emotions with an experience you add more value to that experience and burn it deeper into your brain circuitry. If you employ your emotions in your visions of the future, you will add value to that vision, in your mind's eye, and further increase the odds of noticing things in your daily environment that might take you down that road. It's not like there will be a big flashing neon sign saying 'DO THIS', but you will find yourself giving different opportunities more thought, or a second look. Of course, anytime you try to accomplish something new you will need to take some risk. You can't act on any opportunity without putting something at stake. Usually, the bigger the opportunity, the bigger the risk, but that is part of life's exciting experiment.

Denis Waitley, the former director of sports psychology for the U.S. Olympic team, teaches that experience allows you to see opportunity, whereas inexperience causes you to see only risk and fear. But how can you act on opportunity with confidence and positive expectations before you get the experience? One way is to do the dress rehearsal in your mind and discuss it with supportive people. Go through the situation over and over again before you actually need to face it. You can practice controlling your emotions using the same brain circuits that will be in control during the real thing and get them ready to perform when called upon. Professional and Olympic athletes use visualization all the time to perform perfectly in their mind before they need to perform in reality. In fact, visualizing physical actions, as in sports psychology, goes beyond activating circuits within the brain that control movement. This technique actually activates the neural circuits that leave the brain and go down to the muscles that you would use to accomplish the actions you are visualizing. It's really an amazing technique for preparing for all kinds of experiences, not just sports. Visualization will give you a sense of control and confidence, because, if you've been there before (even in your mind), there is less opportunity to be surprised. This preparedness, can help reduce stress and improve performance in nearly any situation.

Stay Out Of Stress

It's not too hard to understand how emotional state and cognitive ability couple very tightly. Your cognitive focus affects your mood, including what you find positive and exciting, or what you find stressful or risky. Your mood, in return, affects your moment-to-moment cognitive performance, including the things you pay attention to, remember, and learn; and the creativity and confidence with which you approach challenges.

Have you ever tried to concentrate on something when you are feeling stressed out? You can't do it. This is why people who can stay calm in a crisis do so much better. You just can't think clearly when you're in a panic. There are physiological reasons for this. When you're stressed out your body releases hormones that help you deal with that stressor. In the cave man days stress usually meant you had to escape a dangerous situation, like a lion, right then and there. It didn't mean worrying about whether or not you will owe on your taxes.

These 'life or death' situations divert energy from your 'pondering' skills, to your 'escape skills'. No reason to ponder the meaning of life when you have a tree to climb so you don't get impaled by a charging rhinoceros. Stress hormones actually shut down certain higher processing centers in your brain and divert that energy to parts of your nervous system required for fight or escape (the fright, flight or fight response). Back then, it was all for our benefit, but today we experience so much more psychological stress (whether real or imagined) that this

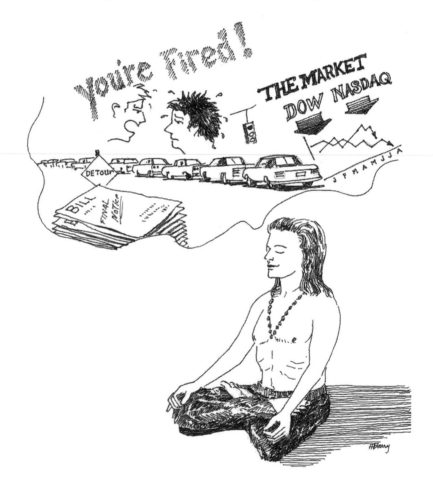

"Relaxation exercise can help take the edge of the daily stressors in your life and reduce the activation of brain circuits that contribute to stressful feelings."

response doesn't serve us so well. We tend to activate our stress response at low or moderate levels in many common, daily experiences. We deal with annoying bosses and co-workers, we get stuck in traffic when we're in a hurry, we deal with (or maybe are) over-zealous youth sports parents, and all the other stuff modern life throws our way. All of this leads to decreased emotional stability and decreased cognitive performance.

It's also much more difficult to focus when you're in a bad mood, or feeling depressed. In these mood states, you may find your mind in an internal battle. You may want to focus on finishing that proposal that's due tomorrow, but your mind won't let go of that jerk who flipped you off on your way into the office this morning. Again, your emotional state is controlling your cognitive and reasoning abilities in the moment.

The more you can control your mood states, the better you can perform in all others aspects of brain fitness. The mental activities that you participate in (whether deliberately or not) have a dramatic affect on your emotional health. We spent the last chapter discussing how using specific brain circuits make them stronger. This goes for emotional circuits as well. If you are constantly engaging in activities that stress you out or put you in a bad mood, guess what, you will make it easier and easier to enter that mood state. Likewise, the more you activate brain circuits that control positive emotions, the easier it will be to return to those mood states.

Like anything else, practice makes permanent (or semi-permanent). You can't just change your drive to enter certain mood states overnight. Your brain circuits take time to adjust, rewire, and strengthen the new circuitry you are trying to build. You also can't change by simply wanting to change, while continuing to do the same things you have always done. The best definition of insanity is "doing the same things you have always done and expecting different results."

In addition to general positive thinking, discussed above, there are different systematic mental techniques to focus your mind and achieve a desired emotional state. It is beyond the scope of this book to cover all of those, but we will visit a few that have some good scientific data behind them. Sometimes people use mental techniques to maintain their emotional and physical health, even if they don't have a problem. Other times, mental health professionals employ these techniques to help people deal with depression, anxiety or other mood related disturbances.

Live In The Present

One technique that has been gaining popularity over the last several years, for use in sickness or in health, is mindfulness. This technique originated in Buddhism and has slowly gained acceptance in western medicine. To be clear, even though mindfulness came from Buddhism, you don't have to be Buddhist to use it. In fact, it doesn't matter whether or not you have any religious inclination.

Jon Kabat-Zinn is a biomedical scientist trained at Massachusetts Institute for Technology who played a large role introducing mindfulness to the western world in the late 1970s. Today, the University of Massachusetts offers certification in mindfulness training to clinicians and other practitioners. In a nutshell, mindfulness is 'paying attention' and 'being in the present on purpose'. If you're a Star Wars fan, you can liken it to the Jedi mindset. Of course, no one suggests that mindfulness will help you tap into 'The Force' to control objects with your mind. However, you can tap into yourself to control your own experiences. Mindfulness is essentially observing your own thoughts and experiences without judgment. Practitioners recognize their thoughts as just thoughts. They understand that their thoughts and feelings may be inaccurate and not represent the truth.

For example, let's say your boss just gave you a deadline at work and you don't feel that you have the time to meet it. This may instantly create stress and a feeling of being overwhelmed. If you were regularly using mindfulness, you might recognize that feeling as something your mind just created based on the information you received. You would view the feeling as just that, a feeling or thought, but not validate it as accurate. You would be able to acknowledge the stress but then let it go and attend to the task, which is to work on meeting the deadline. The feeling of stress itself will not help you do what you need to do. In fact, it will probably delay you or get in the way. Your initial interpretation that there is no way you can do what is being asked, might not be the truth. Once you begin the project, you might find that you will complete it easier than you think. Practicing mindfulness allows you to reserve judgment on the accuracy of your thoughts and feelings and just observe them for what they are, products of your mind.

Learning mindfulness programs vary, but typically employ an eight-week or so training program, often coupled with some type yoga or Tai Chi. When learning mindfulness, meditation is used to provide a 'framework' to get acquainted with the technique in a quiet environment. Meditation does not have to be some weird thing where you sit with your palms up in an incensed filled room uttering mystical chants. Meditation simply is a period of reflection where you can focus without distraction from the outside world. Students learning mindfulness are encouraged to practice 30 minutes or so a day to become comfortable with the technique.

Mindfulness training often begins with a body scan, in which the practitioner lays down in a comfortable position and focuses sequentially on each part of their body. They are instructed to feel the contact of each body part with the ground or mat, the weight and feeling of clothing, the temperature of each part, etc. However, they are also instructed to acknowledge each feeling then let it fade and move on. They are supposed to disconnect any thoughts of the past or future and experience everything completely in the present. This helps train the mind to experience the present moment for what it is, with no judgment, prior context or preconceived expectations. The cool thing about mindfulness is that once learned, it is not something you need to find extra time to do. Once mastered, you can use mindfulness when you're up and walking around or going about your normal day.

You can use mindfulness to improve several aspects of your own brain fitness. A major focus that people use mindfulness for is stress reduction. Many studies document the success of mindfulness-based stress reduction programs. Additionally, studies show success of using mindfulness techniques to improve empathy for other people and strengthen the quality of romantic relationships. All of these probably work because mindfulness can improve your own emotional intelligence by increasing self-esteem and social skills.

Beyond everyday life, mindfulness has clinical value in treating several mental and physical health issues. Not surprisingly, based on our prior discussion, mindfulness can be useful for treating mood disorders. Several studies have tested mindfulness approaches to helping improve bipolar disorder, anxiety disorders and depression, including reducing suicidal thoughts. Limited data also show value for using mindfulness to reduce aggressive behavior and improve ADHD in adolescents and in adults. This doesn't mean that all mental health patients respond to mindfulness training or that it is a cure-all for mental health disorders. However, at least for some people, mindfulness appears to be an effective treatment, either alone or in combination with other therapies. In fact, some patients who are not responsive to standard pharmaceutical treatments are more responsive to mindfulness therapies. The beauty of this technique is that there are no side effects.

Other disorders of a more physical nature can also show positive response to mindfulness training. In one study researchers evaluated using mindfulness in older women with chronic back pain and found a significant improvement in pain tolerance. Another study looked at the affect of mindfulness in dealing with fibromyalgia with similar results in pain tolerance, coping skills and general complaints. Finally, the technique has improved the quality of life of patients who suffer from a traumatic brain injury. Although mindfulness does not reverse the symptoms of all of these disorders, it helps patients deal with their problems to reduce the stressful component of having an illness.

Importantly, research documents mindfulness success for all age-ranges, from children and high-school students to working and retired adults. Based on our previous discussions, it's really no surprise. When you use your brain in a deliberate way, you can improve it. We'll visit a few more aspects of mindfulness in the next chapter in the context of mind-body connections. There's some cool data on how this technique can actually affect the health of your physical body, in addition to your mind.

Cognitive Control

Another technique, which has over 40 years of history in the psychiatry field, is cognitive behavioral therapy. Unlike mindfulness, cognitive behavioral therapy, or CBT, is mostly used in the clinical setting. Psychiatrists originally developed it to treat depression. However, they have since applied it to a host of other mental health concerns. CBT is relevant to our discussion on emotional intelligence because about 15% or 1 out of 7 people in the United States battle depression at some point in their life. It is a common problem. Depression is also intertwined with other health problems and with cognitive disorders like Alzheimer's disease.

Decades ago, sufferers kept depression hidden for the fear of public ridicule, but today there is no reason to hide from it. Even though some stigma may remain around a diagnosis of depression, we understand enough about the illness today to know that this should not be the case. Sometimes you can do everything right and still go through bouts of depression for many different reasons. If you or someone you know shows signs of depression, seek professional help because there is a lot that we can do to help them.

CBT has shown robust success at treating depression in children and adults for many years and keeping depression from recurring for people in remission. Additionally, CBT has proven highly useful to treat panic attacks and social phobias and has shown moderate success treating marital distress, anger, chronic pain and insomnia. All of these can put a damper on your emotional intelligence and your overall level of brain fitness.

As with mindfulness, CBT asks you to be aware of your thoughts and feelings. However, the big difference is that mindfulness asks you not to judge your thoughts, but just to acknowledge them and let them go. CBT, on the other hand, asks you to recognize negative or destructive thoughts (by judging them as so) and replace them with positive thoughts. Patients undergoing CBT are often asked to keep a diary of significant events, thoughts and feelings. They are asked to challenge any disempowering beliefs and replace them. For example, CBT patients should catch themselves whenever they find themselves feeling inadequate or incapable and replace those images of themselves with empowering and capable ones. Often, CBT gets back into the realm of self-help and personal development discussed in the earlier part of this chapter.

In the end, all these techniques play back into the idea that you want to use your mind to activate brain circuits that make you feel stable, powerful and capable. At the same time, you want to reduce the activation of circuits that lead to uncontrollable stress, disempowerment or feelings of inadequacy. In essence, you want to make the positive circuits stronger and the negative circuits weaker. Sounds simple, but with persistence and commitment it can have a huge impact on your EQ and your over-all sense of well-being.

Moving On

The next chapter will focus much more deeply on the mind-body connection and just how much power your mental thoughts have over your physical health and the performance of many body functions. How do your personal beliefs benefit or hinder your health?

Let's explore that question a little more.

CHAPTER 12

MIND OVER MATTER

Mind Control Of Your Physical Intelligence

"What the mind dwells upon, the body acts upon".
- Denis Waitley (author, sports psychologist and speaker)

As we discussed in previous chapters, your brain exerts a lot of control over the rest of your body. It's not too difficult to make the connection on how topics of the last two sections, nutrition and exercise can benefit the body and the brain. However, the topic of this chapter, mental activity and physical intelligence, may seem a little less intuitive. Yet there are ample data supporting roles for many different types of mental activities (some of which we've already discussed in other contexts) on how your body functions. In this chapter, we'll focus on how your very thoughts affect the response of other body systems. This discussion applies to health and disease. We'll discuss how your thoughts can keep you healthier and how, sometimes, they can help you recover from different diseases or disorders. Your mind is an incredible thing. We know that your thoughts affect how well your immune system fights infections, how much your brain releases chemicals to fight pain, and even how responsive you will be to standard medical treatments. In fact, entire fields of science are now devoted to understanding these powers of the mind. The field of psychoneuroimmunology (say that five times fast) is devoted to understand how the mind (psycho-neuro) controls the immune (-immun) system and vice-versa. The field of psychoneuroendocrinology focuses on understanding how thoughts (psycho-neuro) control the release of brain and body hormones (-endocrin) and how those hormones feedback to control thoughts.

Using your mind to control your body functions, as it applies to maintaining health or improving physical ailments, really falls into the realm of mind-body medicine. Just a couple of decades ago, the western medical community poo-poo'd this term as some funky mystical approach that lay outside the realm of 'real treatment'. However, today the western world has made significant strides to come around and mind-body approaches have gained popularity in our culture and in our medical practices (yes, even outside of California). In fact, in 1999 the U.S. government earmarked $10 million of the National Institutes of Health budget specifically to study "Mind-Body Interactions and Health".

The Power Of Belief

Mental activities that affect physical health mostly fall within different types of meditative practices and belief systems. There are many types of meditative practices with proven physical benefits, which will be the focus of the latter half of this chapter. However, simply having a positive attitude and a belief in what you are doing can have dramatic effects on your physical health as well. These attitudes and beliefs all fall under the umbrella of mental activity because the thoughts you think and the conversations you have with yourself are activating brain circuits that contribute to your overall mental activity. This chapter will help you achieve positive results from using mental activity to your advantage. As part of that objective, you should be aware of the negative possibilities of damaging mental activities or destructive thoughts, since these can contribute to stress and disease. The United States estimates $17 billion a year of lost productivity from stress-related disorders, making the point that getting a handle on your own mental activities is crucial for your physical health.

In the first half of this chapter, we'll give you several examples of how positive and negative thoughts affect your overall physical health. In the second half of the chapter, we'll point you down some roads that can help you spend more time on the positive side to improve your overall physical intelligence. We'll start off with a discussion on the power of belief and then return to some specific activities.

We are only beginning to understand the power of your mind and its control over your physical body. However, one thing is certain. Beliefs play a huge role in your mind's powers. Studies looking at the 'placebo effect', underscore this. A placebo is a pill or other type of treatment that has no active medical benefit in and of itself. Originally, we used placebos along with test treatments (like new drugs) to see whether the new treatment worked better than 'nothing' (in quotes because as we'll see below, nothing may not be nothing at all). Essentially, with a placebo treatment, researchers attempt to do everything the same as in the real treatment with the exception of giving the active drug itself. For example, when testing a new blood pressure medicine, half the test subjects will get the real medicine and the other half will get a pill that looks, tastes and smells the same, but has no drug in it.

Researchers must use placebo control groups because in most studies, as we're about to find out, people taking only the placebo show significant improvement. So in order to evaluate the beneficial effects of a new drug, it must be compared to the benefits of a placebo in order to make sure the drug works better than the placebo control. Just believing that you are taking something that might make you better is, in many cases, enough to have a beneficial effect. Although the magnitude of the placebo effect is still under debate, many studies estimate it around 30%, meaning one out of three people get better simply because they know they might be in the real drug treatment group. In the first placebo controlled trial, published in 1801, the author, John Haygarth, concluded, *"An important lesson in physic is here to be learnt, the wonderful and powerful influence of the passions of the mind upon the state and disorder of the body"*.

Sometimes the power of belief can also come into play to make an actual drug treatment better. For example, painkillers delivered by doctors in a clinic work better if the patient knows they are getting them and the doctor tells them they should feel better. As opposed to patients receiving painkillers through an i.v. in their arm where a computerized pump delivers the medicine at times unknown to the patient. Patients that know they are receiving pain medications feel better than those treated without their knowledge do. This also relates to the power of expectations. When researchers tell study volunteers that they are receiving a powerful painkiller, they feel much better than those told that they might be receiving either a painkiller or a placebo. This is true even if all volunteers are actually only receiving placebo. When people expect to have a positive response to a treatment, they often will, even if the treatment has no medicinal value. This creates a difficulty in defining medicinal value, since patients improve with placebo, shouldn't that be considered medicinal value as well?

It's clear that beliefs, expectations and desires, affect your results. If you're in pain and you believe a specific treatment will help you, you have a greater chance of benefiting from that treatment. This all relates back to mental activity because the placebo effect itself appears to work by activating and inactivating specific brain circuits that control your perceptions. Researchers use brain-imaging studies to try to understand the different brain circuits involved in the placebo effect. While there is much work left to do, they have identified many brain circuits and systems that play a role in different aspects of the placebo effect. When it comes to placebo treatment of pain, the opioid system seems to play a large role. Opioids (sometimes called endorphins) are involved in pain control and is the system that drugs like heroin or morphine interact with to cause their 'feel good' effects. Patients given placebos for pain therapy show increased activity in the pain controlling opioid circuits in their brains. What this research suggests is that your own beliefs and expectations can activate brain centers to produce a real physiological response that goes beyond mere perceptions.

These concepts are highly relevant to using mental activity to control your PQ, given our previous discussions on how the activities of brain circuits can strengthen or weaken those circuits and influence their future performance. The stronger your beliefs and expectations, the more likely you are to use brain circuits that further strengthen those beliefs, which in turn, can control the outcome of future challenges. To be clear, this can be good or bad. If you are someone who believes that you will have a positive outcome, you are more likely to get the result that you want. On the other hand, if you continually believe that you will have a negative outcome, guess what, you are more likely to perceive that as well.

Don't Give Me That Attitude! Unless It's Good.

Beyond your perception of a given situation, some interesting studies show that your attitude can control your body's physical responses. This moves past the usual 'glass half full' or 'half empty' analogy. Studies have looked at the power of positive attitude to control susceptibility to getting a common cold or the flu. Researchers recruited study volunteers by interviewing people over the phone to determine whether they had a positive or negative attitude. Now, everyone has good days and bad days so the researchers interviewed the same people several times over a two-week period to give them an accurate measure as a positive or negative person. After the ratings were complete, the study volunteers came into the clinic where they knew that researchers would infect them using a nasal spray containing the virus for either a common cold or the flu. Researchers then quarantined the volunteers (in separate areas for either the flu or a cold).

For the next several days, the volunteers reported the severity of their symptoms and researchers tracked their mucus production, fever, and other objective symptoms. Researchers also took blood samples to measure virus levels to determine the success of the infection. Now, you would expect those with a negative outlook to complain more about the degree of their symptoms, including muscle aches, joint pain, chills, etc., and that's exactly what researchers found. Positive people actually had less measurable symptomology, including less mucus production, lower fevers and other objective measures. But here's the interesting part. It was more than perception. Their blood tests also showed lower rates of successful infection from the common cold bug than did the negative attitude folks! This study demonstrated the power of having a positive outlook and expecting the best, regarding controlling your own physical health. Even though researchers exposed both groups to equal doses of viral infection, the positive attitude group did not get as sick as the negative attitude group, probably through having a healthier immune response.

Another interesting study took a different spin on how positive beliefs interact with other healthy behaviors to provide you with greater benefit. In the last section, we detailed the benefits of exercise and physical activity on brain function. One interesting study showed how a positive belief makes the benefits of exercise even better. Researchers recruited 84 female housekeepers from several different hotels and explained to half of them how their jobs met the surgeon general's daily recommendations for exercise. Study organizers gave specific examples of how the housekeeper's cleaning activities were physically rigorous and good for their overall health and cardiovascular system. Researchers then observed the housekeepers, along with those who weren't given this information, for the next four weeks. What they found surprised them. Although the housekeepers behavior did not

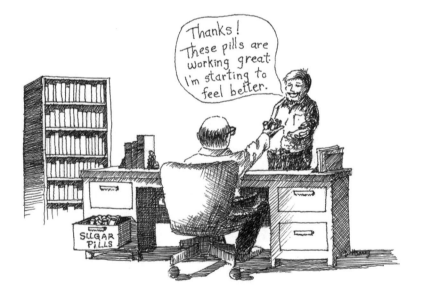

"Believing that you are taking medication that will help a health problem can, sometimes, be as powerful as real medication itself."

change in either group, the health of those 'in the know' improved. The housekeepers educated on the benefits of their profession's physical activity lost weight (mostly body fat), reduced their blood pressure, and lowered their hip-to-waist ratios and body mass index. This provides another strong example of the power of belief.

So here's a question. If the placebo effect is so strong, why not just convince yourself that lounging in front of the TV eating chips all day is beneficial for your health? Maybe we should just convince our kids that all those cookies and cartoons are good for their brains? Well, in this case you would have two opposing forces struggling against each other, so that's not likely to work. Believing things that have no real affect are good for you, is one thing. Believing that things that are bad for you, are actually good for you, is something entirely different. If you were truly able to convince yourself that unhealthy habits were actually healthy, you may be able to reduce the ill effects of those habits. But it's unlikely you would actually be able to reverse them. The powers of your mind work best when they synergize with your body chemistry, not try to fight them.

Methods Of Mind Control

Now we'll turn our attention to actual activities you can do to increase your own control of your mind and make it easier to use positive beliefs and attitudes to improve your physical intelligence. One of the most common and well-studied approaches is using meditation techniques. Before we get into that, however, let us dispel some myths. Meditation is not some weird, hairy fairy, approach to tap into mystical hidden powers. Meditation is simply a way to remove yourself temporarily from the hectic pace of life and pay attention to your own thoughts. Some believe that meditation does indeed put you in connection with a universal power. Whether or not that is true is not the point of this discussion. Like we mentioned in previous sections, 'how' something works doesn't really change the fact that it works. We know that meditative practices have health benefits and that is what we will focus on. If you never take time to stop and reflect, chances are your environment and your situation will dictate what you think – essentially controlling your mental activities. You get caught up in the rat-race, the daily grind, running from one place to the next to make sure you get everything finished. Meditation (and there are many different types) is a way to take back control of your own mental activities so that you can use your mind purposefully.

Meditative techniques come from Western and Eastern cultures, dating back centuries. You can find mediation references in early writings from Christian, Jewish, Islamic, Hindu and Buddhist literature. The major types of meditation receiving the most current use and research attention stem from Transcendental meditation, Mindfulness meditation, meditative prayer and different kinds of Yoga (mostly Hatha Yoga in the Western world). Each of these have their own unique approaches and have been tested in the treatment of various physical ailments. Studies have evaluated the ability of meditation to treat asthma, cardiovascular illnesses, anxiety and depressive disorders, epilepsy, sleep problems, stress, pre-menstrual and menopause symptoms, drug dependence, multiple sclerosis, tinnitus (ringing of the ears), pain due to arthritis, and psoriasis. Although meditation does not always work, there seems to be a significant clinical benefit for many people. We'll discuss below, the arguments for benefits of different types of meditation for specific ailments, but one commonality across all studies appears clear. There is very little down-side to using these techniques (aside from a consistent time commitment) and no real evidence for negative side effects. Any adverse responses to meditative approaches seem to be rare. When's the last time you saw a drug commercial on TV that could claim that?

Some of the techniques we will discuss below (e.g. Yoga and Tai Chi) require both physical and mental activity. It's impossible to say for sure which of these components provides the greatest benefit, when in fact, it may be both. One of the major themes throughout this entire book is the futility of attempting to separate the mind from the body. So although we could have discussed these techniques in the physical activity section as well, we decided they fit nicely into the context of mental activity – but it doesn't really matter.

It is beyond the scope of this book to provide a detailed program for any of these techniques. We simply want to alert you as to the science behind their health benefits so you can consider pursuing them for your own purpose. Readers interested in these approaches are encouraged to seek the help of a licensed fitness instructor as well as the advice of your physician as to whether or not these are viable options in your physical state of health.

Yoga

There are various types of Yoga, ranging from physical poses to pure meditation. Hatha Yoga is most common in the Western world, and focuses primarily on the physical activity of the movements and poses. However, this form of Yoga employs significant concentration and deliberate movement that places it into the realm of mental activity as well. Indian practitioners originally used Hatha Yoga in as training for holding poses utilized by deeper meditative practices.

However, several studies show that Hatha Yoga alone is effective for improving the brain's control over the body when considering both general health and various disease states.

From a general health perspective, there is ample evidence that Hatha Yoga helps people reduce stress and anxiety and increases their sense of well-being. As we discussed *Neural Nugget #4, Stressing Out*, this alone will have health benefits. As far as actual use as a treatment for specific diseases, there are some data on this as well. Studies show benefits of Hatha Yoga for improving blood sugar control and reducing total cholesterol in type II diabetics, a disease that is extremely prevalent in today's developed nations. Other studies show reduction of pain and increased mobility in seniors with osteoarthritis or musculoskeletal disease. Given that these are the leading cause of disability in people over age 65, this is highly relevant to a large percentage of the population. Hatha Yoga also improves lung and heart function in patients with cardiopulmonary disease. Finally, some interesting studies show benefits of Hatha Yoga at helping people recover from drug addictions. It's likely that Yoga practitioners receive many other health benefits as well, but these are the ones with the most scientific support at the current time. It will be interesting to see how Yoga incorporates itself into western society as more and more medical doctors consider alternative health approaches in their clinical practices.

Tai Chi Chuan

Another active research area centers on the utility of Tai Chi Chuan in the maintenance of health and the treatment of disease. The earliest reference to Tai Chi Chuan (which we will abbreviate to Tai Chi from this point on) comes from the Chen family in 1820s China. Although there are many styles of this 'soft' martial art, the most popular in Western cultures is that of slow deliberate movements. Some refer to this form as meditation in motion, because of the focus on a calm mind and deliberate actions. Tai Chi is especially well suited to the aging population because of its relatively mild physical stress. The first widespread recognition of Tai Chi's positive role in health dates back to the early 20th century. Since that time, many people with no interest in the martial art component began to practice Tai Chi for its health benefits. If you have an interest in taking up Tai Chi, it shouldn't be difficult to find a qualified instructor in your area.

Beyond an established role in maintaining general health, research investigating the legitimacy of Tai Chi in treatment of disease has proven positive in many cases. Several studies show that Tai Chi is effective at reducing blood pressure to control hypertension and could be an adjunct therapy to standard treatments. Related to this benefit, Tai Chi is also useful for stroke recovery and rehabilitation. This is probably in part due to its ability to reduce blood pressure, a major risk factor for stroke, but also due to Tai Chi's role in improving balance and mood. The physical movements of Tai Chi likely contribute to its ability to improve balance, which is a major benefit for older people since injuries from falling are a significant problem, especially following a stroke. However, the mental aspects of focused movements will also strengthen brain circuits that control muscle movements, improving balance and coordination. Again, attempting to separate the mental and physical aspects of these benefits are impractical.

Research has also focused on the benefits of Tai Chi for boosting immune function. One study evaluated the role of Tai Chi to help people with HIV infection maintain a healthier immune system. As HIV infection progresses it wipes out the body's immune response, rendering the patient less capable of fighting off other infections. Tai Chi appeared to help maintain the viability of immune function in AIDS patients, potentially contributing to improved health and longevity. Other interesting studies found that Tai Chi improved the immune systems response to flu or shingles vaccinations. Vaccinations work by presenting your immune system with a small piece of an infectious germ so that your body can take note of what that specific germ 'looks like', without the danger of infection. Then if your immune system ever sees the real germ in the future, it will recognize it much faster and attack it before it can spread. Without vaccination, your body may also fight the germ off, but it will take more time and potentially allow the germ to do some damage before your immune system can mount an effective attack. Research has shown that people practicing Tai Chi boosted their immune system's arsenal against the flu and shingles in combination with a vaccination. Whereas people vaccinated who weren't practicing Tai Chi just had the normal response.

Other studies show the benefits of Tai Chi at improving functionality and reducing pain related to osteoarthritis and improving bone density in postmenopausal women. However, some of these studies showed no effect. Overall, the data still seem weak regarding the ability of Tai Chi to help arthritic or bone density problems. But, given the lack of side effects or adverse reactions, it may be worth a shot. After all, none of the studies showed that Tai Chi actually made these conditions any worse, and if you feel you get good results, then why not continue?

Mindfulness

We already discussed mindfulness techniques in the last chapter in the context of emotional health. Several studies also support this technique as having benefits for physical health. It's likely that the way mindfulness improves emotional health and physical health are highly related, perhaps even identical. When clinicians use mindfulness, they typically do so in the context of a structured 'mindfulness based stress reduction' therapy. The 'stress reduction' part is likely a key component of why this approach works, for improvements in both emotional and physical health.

It's difficult to separate mindfulness from other forms of purposeful mental activity because mindfulness training often involves some form of gentle yoga and other relaxation techniques. Regardless of how mindfulness programs work, they appear to have clinical benefits in aiding the treatment of various illnesses, especially those involving the function of the immune system. Studies in women with breast cancer or men with prostate cancer show that mindfulness improves immune system function, which helps your body fight the invasive cancer cells. Similar studies also show that mindfulness reduces blood pressure, reduces blood hormones that elevate stress, improves coping skills, and generally improves perceived quality of life.

A potential advantage to Mindfulness Based Stress Reduction is the fact that there is a standardized program that has been delivered and tested in clinical settings in hundreds of studies. The other techniques discussed above (like Yoga and Tai Chi), certainly have repeatedly demonstrated their value in improving health. However, there are so many variations it's difficult to say what the best approach is for any given illness. If you are simply trying to maintain general health, it makes sense to do whatever you most enjoy. However, if you are actually working with a physician to treat an illness there may be benefit to using a structured program. In this day and age, physicians should at least be somewhat familiar with alternative medicine approaches and open to discussing them with you as an add-on or stand-alone treatment option.

Moving On

In the next chapter, we'll get into mental workouts to improve cognitive function. This is really the central theme of many emerging 'brain fitness companies' attempting to create software to train your brain and keep your mind sharp. How well do they work?

CHAPTER 13

USE IT TO IMPROVE IT

Mental Activities For Cognitive Fitness

"It is not enough to have a good mind; the main thing is to use it well."

- Rene Descartes, circa 1630 (philosopher and mathematician)

This chapter focuses on the central theme of the emerging 'Brain Fitness Industry', which is a mental workout to keep your cognitive mind fit. At the time of this writing all kinds of software products are hitting the market to cater to aging baby boomers and their fears of memory loss and cognitive decline. While this is a legitimate concern for our aging society and there are several evidence-based approaches to fight it (as is the topic of this entire book), there seem to be many products simply exploiting fears. In this chapter, we'll provide an overview as to which types of mental activities have data supporting their benefit for cognitive health, which make sense but still need some investigation, and which lack any support at all. As we've said before, it's arrogant to dismiss the validity of something simply because we don't understand how it works and some current brain fitness products may fit into this category. Brain training approaches are emerging too quickly today for quality science to test and support them. This does not mean that they don't work. It just means that we don't yet know if they work or not. However, buyers should be aware that some marketers hopping on the brain fitness bandwagon are making fairly unlikely and ungrounded claims as to the cognitive benefits of their products. In addition, we believe there is great potential to help people develop a reserve for their aging years, and as we've mentioned, the sooner you start, the better.

When it comes to improving cognitive function, you can divide goals and approaches into a few categories. First, you can strive to improve function to above normal abilities at any age, young or old. This would be in the realm of performance enhancement. From a data perspective, achieving super-normal function is difficult but potentially achievable, depending on how you look at it. We'll get into those data and methods below but the reader should be aware that this field is wrought with snake-oil approaches. People in a competitive environment, like corporate executives, athletes or combat soldiers, are most likely to seek this type of brain development, and there is no shortage of tools for sale promising to get you there. However, some basic, long-term approaches can help keep you at your cognitive best.

Second, you can strive to prevent cognitive decline as you age. This includes maintaining your memory and reasoning powers, at or near the levels that you enjoyed as young adults. These types of prevention-based approaches to reduce cognitive decline as you age carry the most evidence for support. There are several studies supporting the notion that the degree to which you use your intellectual powers in your young adult to middle aged years affect the health at which your brain ages. We'll spend some time discussing those approaches in this chapter.

Finally, your goal may be to recover lost function. This includes using mental workouts to reclaim normal function after you already notice that you've experienced some decline.

Maybe your memory isn't as good as it used to be, the time it takes you to process information and respond is a little slow, or your reasoning abilities seem a little dull. You'd like to reclaim some of those skills and sharpen the knife, so to speak. With some work and tenacity you probably can. Understand though, that the goal of recovering lost cognitive function is a little more difficult. It's easier to prevent loss in the first place than to recover it once you go down an ailing road. As the old adage says, "an ounce of prevention is worth a pound of cure". However, data suggest that you can recover some lost function in your older years, and we'll soon discuss that as well. All of these approaches relate to boosting cognitive fitness, but for different reasons and with different goals. As we go through this chapter, we encourage you to keep that in mind relative to your own needs and desires.

Approaches to improve, maintain or recover cognitive function come in many forms. Some are tools you use for the explicit purposes of improving specific skills, like memory, reaction speed, vocabulary, pattern recognition, creativity or reasoning. This is the crux of the emerging brain fitness software industry, which is putting out more and more tools, attempting to help improve these specific skill sets. Other approaches include daily experiences, educational level, commitments to life-long learning or social support networks. You may engage in these without the expressed goal of improving cognitive function, but many of them will have that beneficial effect anyway!

Performance Enhancement

Performance enhancement for cognitive function comes in several forms. There are many pharmacological (legal and illegal; we assume you are aware of the big drug-testing debate

216 BrainFit For Life

for the 1994 spelling-bee competition) approaches to enhancing performance on the spot, but we are not interested in those. Some of the reasons for using these approaches are legitimate, like short-term military use in field operations. After all, what good is it to focus on life-long health when the most important thing is alertness to survive the moment? Other reasons are less legitimate, like cramming for college tests, staying up all night to meet business deadlines, or jacking up your mind to beat your archrival at bridge, pinochle, euchre, or World of Warcraft. However, these are all outside the realm of what we are promoting in this book, which are lifestyle choices to maintain life-long brain health and fitness. So, this section will focus only on cognitive performance enhancement techniques that fit into the framework of sustainable health.

<u>Party On</u>

A research area that is young in regards to performance enhancement, but keeps popping up as extremely important to many other areas of brain health, is social support and social interactions. Socializing is a mental activity requiring a complex array of cognitive tools to interact with other people in behaviorally, emotionally, and socially acceptable ways. A recent study led by University of Michigan researchers looked at the role of social interactions in enhancing cognitive function, in both long-term and short-term studies. First, the research team examined 3,610 people regarding their degree of social interaction and measures of cognitive performance, using the mini-mental state exam (a standard measure of general cognitive health). They found that people with more social interactions had greater performance on the cognitive tests. Interestingly, this result was true for young adults (24 - 41), middle age adults (42 – 64) and older adults (65 – 96). The effect, especially in young adults, suggests that socializing can boost cognitive function above normal performance.

Several other studies have supported roles for social support in emotional, intellectual and physical health, and we have discussed some of these in other parts of this book. However, the U of M research team went a step farther. They also wanted to see if short social interactions could improve cognitive performance right away. This is a very different question than long-term cognitive abilities and applies directly to the topic of this discussion, performance enhancement. The researchers split college students into three groups. The 'social interaction' group spent 10 minutes in a social activity with another person, while the control group watched 10 minutes of a Seinfeld episode. A third group performed mentally challenging activities, like crossword puzzles, reading comprehension, and other mental games. After the 10-minute period, researchers tested volunteers on various cognitive tasks, including processing speed and working memory. Both the social interaction group and the intellectual activities group significantly outperformed the control group, suggesting that even brief periods of socialization can have immediate cognitive performance enhancing effects. Either that or Seinfeld makes you stupid (if this is true, just imagine what reality TV does to you). So maybe before you go into that next important business meeting, you should 'warm up' with a rousing discussion with your buddy from accounting (as long as his or her name isn't Jerry, George, Kramer or Elaine). The main point being, don't sit on the sidelines, get in and play!

Take It To Heart

Beyond the role of socialization, you can also improve your cognitive capacity to learn by beefing up the emotional content of your experiences. This learning enhancement relates back to the function of the hippocampus (along with other parts of the brain), which we discussed in previous chapters. We talked about the hippocampus as playing an important role in learning and memory. One of the reasons it plays this role is because the hippocampus is also involved in deciding what is important to pay attention to in your environment. You constantly need to reevaluate what's going on around you to prioritize what will capture your attention and focus. Most of the time, you do this subconsciously. You ignore background noise from fans while you are having a conversation. You ignore the weight of your body pushing against the chair while you are reading a book. You ignore all the ads running down the side of the web page while you are reading an article (much to advertiser's dismay). In fact, you are ignoring the majority of sounds, smells and sensations most of the time.

However, if you see a sudden movement out of the corner of your eye or hear a sudden noise, you instantly shift your attention to that. This behavior is hard-wired into our brains so that we attend to potentially dangerous situations. Back in the day of walking around the savanna, looking for food, we had to be on the lookout for lions who wanted to make us their next meal. Your brain is wired to pay extra attention to certain things.

One way to engage extra effort from your brain is to attach emotion to your experience. Your brain sees experiences with strong emotions attached to them as more important and worthy of ensuring that a good memory is stored for that experience. A good teacher knows that students learn better when they are having fun, so injecting humor or entertainment into a lesson improves student's retention of the material. Whenever you need to learn something quickly or at a deeper level, try attaching emotion to the learning experience. You can do this by relating it back to emotional times in your own life, happy or sad.

The same may be true for mild stress. Your brain pays attention to stressful experiences because they also carry emotional value. If something is a little stressful, your brain assumes it is probably important. However, the data evaluating mild stress on cognitive performance and memory are controversial. Many studies show that mild stress can enhance learning and memory, while other studies show that mild stress can inhibit memory. Exercise is one type of mild stress (discussed in chapter 9) that has consistent data to improve cognitive function immediately. It gets your heart rate up and activates your 'alertness' centers in your nervous system.

In other cases, it's not really clear why sometimes stress appears to be good and other times not so good for performance enhancement. It probably comes down to the degree of threat that each person feels under any given stressful condition. You are more likely to remember events that happen near the time of a stressor that made you feel a little threatened. I'm sure you remember exactly what you were doing when you heard that the Twin Towers were attacked by airplanes. The brain wants to file experiences surrounding a threatening time to avoid those threats in the future. Sometimes those experiences have nothing to do with the threat, but the brain will associate them anyway. This can actually work against us to cause severe psychological problems after we have experienced traumatic events like war or rape. Memories of those events can be triggered out of context with some smell or sound that was present during the experience.

To sum this section up briefly, a great approach to using mental activity to enhance short-term cognitive performance is to engage in challenging social situations that have both an element of support and an element of risk. In other words, don't put yourself out there so that you are completely unprotected, but at the same time, don't play it too safe. This will keep you on your toes just enough to keep those 'alertness' brain circuits activated without stressing you out so bad that you can't function.

Preventing Decline

One of the most fascinating areas of protecting the brain from intellectual decline is the concept of 'cognitive reserve'. We touched on this in chapter 10, in our discussion of creating multiple brain circuits to achieve certain tasks. Cognitive reserve is a pervasive theory in psychology that says you can build up your brain throughout life. It suggests that you can create 'extra' brain function to pick up the slack as your brain ages. The simplest analogy to explain the concept of reserve is a financial one. If you have just enough money in the bank to make it through the month, you're fine as long as no unforeseen expenses pop up. If that happens, your bank account will take a hit that it can't handle and you'll be in trouble. If, on the other hand, you have several months of 'reserve' in the bank you'll be OK. In either case, your bank account will take the same hit, but if you have the reserve, you can handle it and rebound without any real problems.

The concept of cognitive reserve suggests that you can build up 'extra brain circuits' so that if one circuit takes a small hit (from aging, a minor injury or something else), another circuit can step in to pick up its function. Importantly, this can happen in a way that you don't notice any decline. Let's go back to our road analogy that we used in chapter 10 to drive home this point a little farther. Let's say that you drive the same route to work every day. You know there are other ways to get there but you aren't familiar with those routes because you never use them. Now let's say that your route to work is undergoing road construction. You would just have to deal with the slow traffic and get to work a little slower. Essentially, your commute would become less efficient. Alternatively, let's say that you take different routes to work all the time. You know three or four different ways to get there, like the back of your hand. If one of your routes is undergoing construction, you simply make a turn and use another route, and you do it automatically and with ease. Your commute to work is just as efficient (unless all your routes are blocked).

If you think of these road routes as brain circuits, you can understand the concept of cognitive reserve. If you constantly engage in different activities and learn different approaches or perspectives, you will have multiple solutions with which to approach any given problem. If for some reason, a small brain circuit is damaged (maybe a small stroke or a brief loss of blood supply), you can divert that circuit's job to another circuit that is still healthy, and you won't notice any loss of function. That's the idea behind cognitive reserve. Now let's look at some of the support for that idea and some of the ways to build your own reserve.

The whole concept of cognitive reserve really took hold when researchers noticed that autopsies of elderly people showed Alzheimer's disease in the brain's of some folks who showed no signs of dementia during their life. Some people's brains had taken physical hits from Alzheimer's disease damage, but did not get the symptoms of the disease. Instead, they maintained sharp minds until the end. This suggested that the brain is capable of dealing with disease in some cases, and launched more studies into the theory of cognitive reserve.

One of the most famous studies that looked at these factors, The Nun Study, received national attention when it made the cover of TIME magazine in 2001. This study evaluated (and continues to) 678 Nuns belonging to the School Sisters of Notre Dame. A major advantage of this study is that it follows a group of sisters who were all school teachers, have similar religious backgrounds (and concomitant lifestyles) and who now live in very similar conditions. This is a researcher's dream because many of individual differences that make most human studies difficult just aren't there. All the nuns had similar careers, upbringings and late-life conditions. Yet some

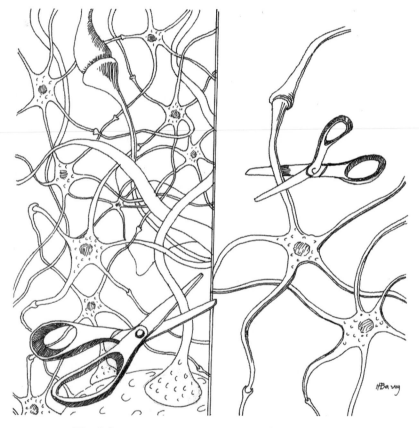

"Building cognitive reserve helps you maintain intellectual function, even if some of your brain circuits become damaged. Focusing on the four cornerstones of brain fitness throughout life can help ward off age-related cognitive decline."

sisters developed cognitive reserve, protecting themselves from dementia, while others did not. We'll get into some strategies for developing and increasing your own cognitive reserve in a minute.

The Nun Study wasn't the first to show a disconnect between Alzheimer's brain pathology and dementia during life, but it provided many other opportunities to ask why this is true. Why do some people escape cognitive decline while others do not, even when the physical degree of Alzheimer's disease in the brain appears to be the same? What leads to the protection of cognitive reserve? We have already covered some of the answers to those questions earlier in this book. We discussed nutritional status in chapter 5 as one factor, especially those linked to cardiovascular health, like folic acid. We discussed exercise and physical activity in chapter 9 as another factor, probably also through improving cardiovascular function and blood supply to the brain. Now, we'll discuss mental activities and experiences that data support as contributing to cognitive reserve in later life.

Keep On Learning

One major factor relevant to mental activity that has a large amount of data to support it as protecting from cognitive decline, is education. Several studies show that having at least a high school education significantly reduces your odds of dementia later in life. A much larger percentage of people, with less than a high school education, have dementia by their mid-seventies than those with at least a high school degree. The gap between educated vs. under-educated people closes as they approach their nineties, but it is still there. Taking a step back, it's probably not the education itself that is the reason for this difference, but what you do with it.

Typically, people with lower education have less intellectually challenging careers for a large part of their life. This leads to less brain-challenges on a day-to-day basis and likely underlies the difference in Alzheimer's rates. That doesn't mean you need a formal education to reduce your odds of dementia. There are plenty of people who didn't finish high school or go to college, but have intellectually challenging careers (e.g. Bill Gates). It's just that when you look at a large group of people, as research studies do, lower education correlates with less intellectual careers on average, and that correlates with higher rates of dementia. So what's the solution? Don't be average. If you did not get much education, you'll just need to work a little harder to either get into an intellectually challenging job or find other ways to work out your brain on a daily basis.

One of the best things you can do, whether you are highly educated or not, is to commit yourself to life-long learning. You should not view education as something you only do when you're young, but should commit to continuing you're education throughout your entire life. Education can take many forms, however. It may be in the form of organized classes that interest you. Maybe you always wanted to learn another language, how to cook Thai food, or understand quantum physics. Education may be in the form of teaching yourself new skills through reading books, listening to audios or watching educational videos. It may also be in the form of tennis lessons, piano lessons or Yoga lessons. It doesn't matter how you choose to continue your education, as long as it challenges your brain to learn new concepts, ideas or skills. Importantly, you should strive for variety and challenges. Don't just focus on things that are easy.

To be clear, all of the data discussed above are correlative. Study after study holds up, showing an association with an active brain in mid- to late-life and reduced risk of dementia. However, researchers can't say for sure that an intellectually active mind is causing the reduced risk – but it sure seems that way.

Recovering Lost Function

As a prescription-minded society, we tend to want to know what the appropriate treatment is for any given ailment. If you have high blood pressure, your doctor will probably prescribe high blood pressure medication. He or she should also attempt to get you to adopt healthy lifestyle changes, but the prescription is the medicine. The same is true for diabetes, heart disease, or insomnia. Each diagnosis will most likely lead to a prescription.

Cognitive decline has no such proven medication (at least not at the time of this writing). However, brain fitness software and cognitive training products are trying to fit that bill. The problem is that cognitive decline is much more complex than many other ailments. Because of that, variety is a key part of the formula to treating it. So far, no cognitive training products have shown real promise at improving global brain function. Many products do improve the specific function they are training you on, like visual pattern recognition, word recall, reaction time, short-term memory capacity, etc. However, these skills mostly apply to doing better in the game itself and may not translate to real-world benefit. So if your goal is to beat your own high score in whatever cognitive game you are using, then it will likely work. But if your goal is to recover your cognitive abilities to go about your daily routines, that's a tougher problem. There are no games out there proven to address all the aspects of brain function needed to pull you out of cognitive decline.

That doesn't mean that current cognitive training software packages are not beneficial. Most researchers believe there is no harm in using the cognitive training games, but realize that it's only a small piece of the overall puzzle. Engagement in many other aspects of life, as we've discussed throughout this chapter and this book, are all part of the brain fitness formula. This means that if you intend to spend your money on cognitive training products, like Nintendo's Brain Age, don't buy into all the marketing hype that goes with it. Everyone wants that magic bullet, that one product or approach that will solve his or her problem. But as we've been promoting, you benefit most by paying attention to all the fundamentals first. If you eat right, get plenty of exercise, sleep well and keep your mind engaged in a variety of activities, then go ahead and have some fun with your brain training software, it may do you some good. Just realize it's not the end-all solution.

However, there is promise on the global training front. A recent study at the University of Michigan showed improvement in 'fluid intelligence' with a specific training protocol. Fluid intelligence is your ability to reason your way to solve problems in areas where you have no prior experience. It's the ability to generalize your knowledge to fit and adapt to new situations, which is what the human brain is so advanced at doing. Researchers in the UM study were able to train volunteers on one cognitive task and get them to improve their performance on a completely different task, which no research had successfully shown before. Working on fluid intelligence is the goal of the brain-fitness software industry and maybe more research on fluid intelligence will eventually get them there.

Another high quality study showed that cognitive training could improve daily living abilities for people over 65.

Researchers wanted to know if they could improve useful cognitive abilities of older adults with specific training programs. They evaluated three different types of training, including memory, reasoning, and processing speed, along with a control group who received no training. Memory training consisted of learning strategies to organize information using visualization and association techniques, in order to memorize word lists, text and other types of materials. Reasoning training involved strategies to find patterns in sequences of letters or pictures. Speed training taught strategies to quickly identify objects with only brief exposure, and to divide attention between tasks. At the end of the training periods, researchers tested volunteers on their improvements in the specific tasks they learned and, importantly, on their improvement in everyday tasks. These included meal preparation, housework, finances, health maintenance, telephone use and shopping.

Each group improved on their specific tasks, supporting the idea that you can get better at the specific cognitive skills you practice. The memory group improved their memory skill; the reasoning group improved their reasoning skills and the speed of processing group improved their cognitive speed. However, only the group trained in reasoning skills showed significant improvement in performing everyday tasks. So in the end, this study supports the possibility of using cognitive training to improve everyday function, but also highlights the fact that not all approaches work.

The good news is that you can improve specific cognitive functions by working directly on these functions. If you want to improve your memory, do some memory training. If you want to improve your processing speed, do some cognitive speed training. The warning message is to be aware of the current limitations of brain fitness software and do your own homework into each product. You can use the resources section in the back of this book to help find some specific advice.

Moving On

In the final section of this book, we'll discuss the ever-important role of sleep in maintaining brain fitness. As much as many people in our society would like to live without sleep, that's not likely to ever happen, regardless in the advancements of our technology. Discover how much sleep you need to optimize your EPIC performance. But first, a recap of mental activities.

MELDING THE MIND MESSAGES

As we've discussed mental activities cover a lot of things, from deliberate practice to hone cognitive skills, to relaxing and de-stressing, to just engaging in life with other people. The types of mental activities that you may want to put more effort into depend on your goals, current state of health, and likes and dislikes. Here we will summarize some key points from this section.

Key Concepts:

- Your brain is always on and the thoughts you think change the physical wiring in your brain.
- Your brain is very 'plastic' and you create new brain cells and new connections throughout life.
- You strengthen the brain circuits you use the most, whether they are positive or negative emotions, thoughts or feelings.
- Beliefs are incredibly powerful things and can activate brain circuits that work to make those beliefs true, whether real or imagined.
- It's easier to prevent cognitive decline by focusing on the four cornerstones than it is to reverse lost cognitive abilities, however you can achieve either to so a degree.
- You can create a 'cognitive reserve' in your brain to help maintain a sharper mind as you age.

Key Action Points:

- Balance new learning with old mastery. This will help you create new connections, while strengthening important existing ones.

- Maintain an active social life. This will help reduce stress and stave off a host of physical and cognitive problems as you age. This can also provide an important support structure for sticking to the four cornerstones.
- Spend some time deliberately living in the present by disengaging from the past or future pressures. This will help you keep perspective and better handle stress.
- Focus on believing in your own abilities and the value of the positive experiences you have. This will help add emotional content to positive experiences and solidify the brain circuits driving them.
- Spend some time learning a calm and mentally focused technique, like Yoga, Tai Chi or Mindfulness. This will help your physical ailments and keep your mind clear of stress.
- Commit to life-long learning by enrolling in a formal class or teaching yourself a new skill, trade or hobby. This will help build up your cognitive reserve and stave off late-life cognitive decline.

The Fourth Cornerstone

Optimal Sleep

CHAPTER 14

SLEEPING YOUR WAY TO THE TOP

Introduction To Sleepy Tools For Brain Fitness

"People who say they sleep like a baby usually don't have one"

- Leo J. Burke (Reverend)

We'll spend one-third of our lives sleeping. But what a waste of time! Lying on our backs, drooling all over our duvet covers while tearing through those dreamland forests with our nasopherangeal chainsaws. Since it is so pointless and is such a waste of time, can't we just avoid it all together and not sleep? Certainly, anyone who has missed a couple nights of solid sleep will immediately see the lunacy in the previous statement. Sleep, in fact, is an exceptionally active and critical part of our lives, especially for our brains. If we're going to spend one-third of our lives asleep, we should probably do a good job of it.

How Much Is Enough?

As with all of the sections of this book, we'll drag the concept of balance back into the spotlight. In order to make our discussion of sleep a little more fluid, we would like to introduce a couple of shorthand concepts. We know that these are generalizations and that the field of sleep-research is much more intricate and sophisticated than the categories that we are about to set up, but this book isn't meant to provide an exhaustive examination of the field of sleep. We'd like to make people aware and interested and supply a base of knowledge that can be expanded upon as needed.

Waking The Sleeping Giant (when he needs another half hour)

We'd like you to think generally about your sleep as either sub-optimal sleep (SOS) or optimal-sleep. We also need to bring to your attention to a couple of concepts used in the field of sleep-research, which are sleep-deficit and sleep recovery. We'll get into these and what they mean for your total brain fitness and EPIC performance as we move through this chapter and section.

We'll be using the shorthand, SOS, for sub-optimal sleep frequently throughout this section. As you can see, this allows us to indulge one of our favorite pastimes, which is creating strings of words that we can collapse into cool acronyms. Under the umbrella of SOS, we would like to group together the categories of sleep loss and sleep disorders. These two types of problems are distinct and will have markedly different treatment approaches, but for the sake of brevity, we will group them for now.

SOS, is a distress call of nautical origins commonly ascribed to mean "Save Our Ship." When you experience Sub-Optimal-Sleep, no matter what the reason, your ship will begin to take on water and you will probably feel the need to send out a distress call. SOS can be a result of behavioral choices, an unwanted side effect of medication or drugs, a specific sleep disorder, or due to some other problem (e.g. mood disorder, restless leg syndrome). For our purposes it will include difficulty falling asleep (e.g. insomnia) and the inability to maintain uninterrupted sleep (a.k.a. fragmented sleep) for whatever reason.

Optimal-sleep, on the other hand is the opposite of SOS. It is where all the planets align, the stars shine, and the heavens smile down on you to meet your optimal sleep needs. You are able to fall asleep quickly and easily, stay asleep throughout the night (non-fragmented sleep), and awake in the morning feeling rested. We deliberately define this in very general terms, since optimal sleep will be a little different for each person, particularly when we talk about the amount of sleep that an individual needs.

To Sleep Or Not To Sleep? Is That The Question?

Another way to ask this would be, "is sleep critical?" This is an important question because many people spend a lot of energy figuring out how to sleep less so they can have more waking hours. Well, how's this for critical? Laboratory rats begin to die if sleep deprived for five days. That's right kids, not snap at the supermarket cashier, not misplace their house keys, not even fall asleep behind the wheel and run into a tree (although all those issues are exacerbated by sleep deprivation as we'll see in a minute). Your biology goes into red-alert and if the problem is not addressed, in extreme cases, death could be the end point.

Does this also happen to humans? We hope that this experiment hasn't been done. However if it were, we would likely see similar consequences. Maybe it would take a little longer but the point is that sleep is absolutely critical. There would certainly be exceptions to the rule. Some people are able to go longer durations without sleep; Special Forces of the armed services and college students on spring break in Tijuana are two examples that readily come to mind.

Scope Of The Problem

A recent Institute of Medicine report on sleep found that between 50 and 70 million Americans "suffer from a chronic disorder of sleep and wakefulness, hindering daily functioning and adversely affecting health." That means approximately one out of six Americans is walking around all bleary-eyed and not functioning at full capacity. Think about the impact that has on productivity at work or school, let alone what kind of danger it produces when someone gets behind the wheel of a car or operates heavy machinery.

About 20% of all serious car crash injuries are a result of driver sleepiness not associated with alcohol. We spend hundreds of billions of dollars each year on medical treatment, over-the-counter drugs, and prescriptions in an attempt to address sleep-related problems. People who suffer from SOS, are less productive, have a greater reliance on health care services, and have elevated risk for injury.

According to a recent Center for Disease Control study examining the sleep patterns from four states (New York, Rhode Island, Delaware, and Hawaii), only approximately 30% of people reported having no nights of SOS over the previous month. That means 70% of the people contacted had at least 1 night of sleep that wasn't completely restful. That's probably not too surprising to you, but wait. It gets better. Only about 30% of the respondents reported having sub-optimal-sleep *totaling* less than one week over the past month. The remaining 40% had more than a total of one week of SOS, which is about 2 nights per week on average. So that's 2 out of 5 people getting poor sleep at least 2 nights per week. Broken down further, approximately 11% of the total respondents reported having SOS every night during the previous 30 nights. EVERY NIGHT! So, 1 of 10 people in this study did not get even one night of restful sleep over a month's time. WOW! That's a substantial chunk of the people that are unable to get the rest that they need. It makes you wonder how long that could continue without leading to other problems; probably not long. It may not surprise you that there is a strong association between mood disorders (e.g. anxiety, depression) and SOS. Imagine how you would feel if you didn't get a good night's sleep for a full month. Maybe you already know.

In some cases, society imposes SOS on people. Approximately 1 out of 5 workers in industrialized countries performs shift-work. This requires them to work, at least partially, during the night and attempt to sleep during the day. In the United States, this amounts to approximately 20 million individuals who have shifted their sleep/wake cycle in order to work. A lot of research has been done on shift-workers and it appears to be a real challenge for people with these types of schedules to maintain optimal levels of sleep.

Too Little, Too Late

Ok, so absolutely no sleep for five days is a drastic experience. But what about losing out on a couple hours here and there? How much can we *cheat* on sleep? What if we just shave off an hour or so a night? Six and a half hours isn't much different than seven and a half hours, is it?

Scientists are finding that this type of sleep deprivation is detrimental as well. Extended periods of losing 1 to 2 hours out of your normal sleep pattern can result in a variety of problems including weight-gain, diabetes, impaired memory performance, altered hormonal patterns, and mood swings (this last one is obvious to most people). According to the Centers for Disease control, the percentage of men and women who sleep less than 6 hours per night has significantly increased over the past 35 years. It may not be such a coincidence that this decrease in sleep behavior parallels the increased rates of obesity in the United States.

In reality, most of us need more sleep, but it is one of the first things we neglect when we are overscheduled. We have more options available to us than ever before, hundreds of high-definition cable channels, endless internet to explore, more to do at work, more to do with the kids. It may be as basic as the general feeling that we should be doing something other than sleeping. That sleep isn't productive, therefore it doesn't deserve any priority. It seems that many people today are looking for 'permission' to get more sleep. Well, we would like to give it to you. As we discuss throughout this section, sleep is productive and you should view it that way.

We'd like to point out, in many cases, especially in older adults, sleep loss is *not* by choice but due to difficulty falling or staying asleep. Insomnia is the most commonly reported sleep problem, however the impact of this condition on general health has been elusive. Researchers have had difficulty showing direct causative links between chronic sleep curtailing (losing a couple hours a night for an extended period of time) and a specific disease. What we do know is that only a few nights of SOS results in unhealthy changes in the physiology and hormone systems of healthy individuals. Stated another way, SOS forces us to make withdrawals from the physical reserves we've worked so hard to build.

Our bodies are very protective of our sleep, so if we experience a night of total sleep deprivation (meaning we don't sleep at all) we will make up for it the following night. But what we have been able to do is trick our bodies out of this protective response by cheating ourselves out of an hour or two every night. Many times this goes unnoticed since we have fancy, and tasty, stimulants to help us get through periods of daytime drowsiness. Numerous energy drinks litter the market, not to mention the designer coffee craze that started back in the early 1990's. So once again we're faced with the role of technology in changing our lives and our health. But in the case of SOS not only do technological advances give us the opportunity to cheat ourselves out of sleep, but we also have readily available ways to work around (chemically) our bodies attempts to tell us that we need to come back into balance. These types of technological changes have not only been associated with decreases in sleep in industrialized nations, but with major changes in the levels of physical activity that we require on a day-to-day basis (see *"The Way We Were"* in chapter 6).

This is an interesting opportunity for digression. If you look at several cultures around the world, and even our own culture before the advent of electricity and related technologies, sleep occurred a couple times a day. The siesta culture of several Latin and Mediterranean countries is one example to consider. They will often take a few hours after lunch for a long nap before returning to work or other tasks of the day. Now overall it might seem like they sleep more than one would during a typical eight-hour stint in the US. But if you do the math, these cultures tend to stay up much later into the night, so overall the amount of sleep works out to be about the same.

In another interesting tidbit, there are historical reports of a common practice of second sleep. Back in the olden-days (prior to electricity) people would work throughout the day, and then when it got dark they would go inside and go to bed. When you live on a small farm in a rural part of, lets say, anywhere, there are only so many stories that Grandpa can come up with to keep everyone entertained. Plus, everyone was probably fairly tired from all the physical activity they were getting on the farm, so in general once people had eaten and things were relatively tidied up, it was time for bed. However, an interesting thing happened. These people would get up in the middle of the night to have a little snack, chat for a bit (no doubt stumble out to the outhouse) and then, after a couple of hours, go back to bed until the morning.

Think about what you would do with your time if you had no electricity, especially if you live at higher latitudes during the winter months. There are stretches where it gets light at 7:30 in the morning and is dark by 5:15, that's not a whole lot of daylight to work with (we know, we live in one of those places). It's also a whole lot of dark time to be sleeping, so you would need to break that up a little. The point of this digression is to highlight the relatively rapid change that many aspects of our lives have experienced in a relatively short amount of time both chronologically (number of calendar years) and biologically (number of generations). These are big changes in a short amount of time.

There is no hard and fast rule in terms of how much people should sleep. The optimal amount of sleep that works for each person will differ slightly, but the underlying rule of balance applies universally. Too little sleep is detrimental to our health and mental well-being. Too much sleep is detrimental to our health and mental well-being. This may sound contradictory but just remember that balance is key in almost every situation that pertains to our bodies and minds. Too much or too little of any given thing can send us out of balance, causing ripples that affect other aspects of our lives.

Setting The Stage(s)

Since sleep is such an important and dynamic part of a full third of our lives, it would be worth talking a little bit about some of the things that happen in our brains when we sleep. Specific parts of our sleep control different physiological functions and these parts are organized into stages. There is still a fair amount of controversy in the sleep research community as to the exact function of specific stages of sleep. But we do know that lack of sleep (overall) adversely affects cognitive, emotional, and physiological performance.

If you thought it was just as simple as lying down and closing your eyes, hold on, we have some ground to cover. Like we mentioned, sleep occurs in stages. There are several distinct phases of sleep during which different physiological processes occur. The two most distinctive phases are REM sleep and non-REM sleep. This has nothing to do with the alternative rock band from Athens Georgia, and everything to do with the reflexive movement of our eyes during this stage of sleep. REM is the acronym for 'Rapid Eye Movement,' originally identified because of the side-to-side eye movement observable under a person's eyelids while they are sleeping. We'll come back to REM sleep in a minute. First, we'll move through the stages of sleep in order they occur, starting with laying our heads down to rest.

Sleep starts in the non-REM phase. Non-REM sleep further divides into 4 stages (1-4) with each increase in number representing a relative increase in the how deeply we sleep; 1 being the lightest sleep and 4 being the heaviest. Throughout the night, REM and non-REM sleep phases will alternate cyclically, and each has its own unique set of behavioral and physiological characteristics including differences in heart rate, brain activity, energy expenditure, muscle contraction and so on. We will explore each of these stages of sleep in the following sections because the time you spend asleep effects what kind of sleep you get, which ultimately feeds back on your cognitive performance.

Sleep is also a progressive progress. The pattern, or cycling, of REM and non-REM sleep changes as we move through the night. The amount of time you spend in REM sleep increases each time you cycle through it and tends to become the longest during the last third of your sleep session. In non-REM sleep, you tend to spend more time in stage-2. In fact, as you move towards the end of your sleep session, stages 3 and 4 become very short, or disappear all together. We will discuss the importance of stage-2 sleep in relation to how sleep affects your metabolism in chapter 16.

After your first cycle of stages 1 – 4 you transition into your first phase of REM sleep. This is the stage of sleep where you experience dreams, and is an essential component of sleep. You can't move directly from an awakened state to REM sleep, unless you have a sleep disorder like narcolepsy. You must travel through non-REM sleep first. Further, the proportion of time spent in REM compared to non-REM sleep is relatively low. So if you're continually interrupted during your sleep it is unlikely that you are accruing necessary levels of REM sleep. Therefore, it is imperative that you give yourselves sufficient opportunity to gain access to REM sleep, and the best approach for this is by giving yourselves permission to sleep and setting aside sufficient time to do so.

In laboratory settings, REM sleep can be specifically disturbed, while allowing other stages of sleep to continue. For some time, researchers believed that disruption of REM sleep resulted in lower learning and memory performance. Studies on learning and memory indicated that this phase of sleep is important for consolidation of memories; in other words, moving them from short-term to long-term storage. However, the role for REM sleep in learning and memory is now fairly controversial in the research community. It's clear that memory consolidation happens during sleep, but nailing down the specific stage responsible is still up in the air. We'll get into the importance of sleep for making memories in chapter 17.

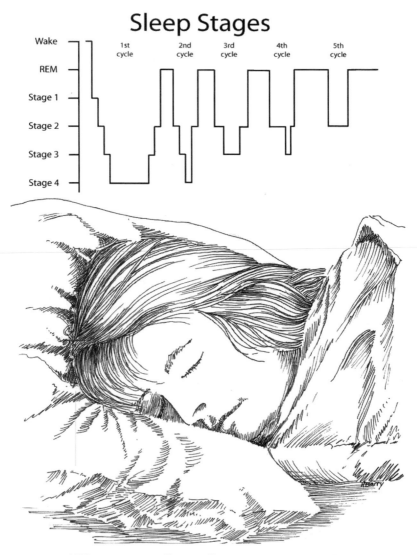

"*Sleep typically adheres to a cyclical and progressive architecture, building throughout the night, This is why it is important to give the construction ample time. Rome wasn't built in a day, and optimal-sleep can't be built in four hours.*"

Sleep And Aging

Sleeping too much generally won't be a problem as we move past our early twenties. People tend to have fewer total hours and lower quality of sleep as they age, even if you account for sleep-loss due to daily responsibilities (e.g. work, family, and so forth). Individuals also tend to become less active as they age, which may influence their sleep patterns, since exercise improves both sleep quality and duration. But we wouldn't advise that you just go out and run a marathon that might result in an irreversible state of sleep, in a manner of speaking.

If you haven't exercised for awhile and are concerned about increasing your physical activity you might consider Tai Chi, which we discussed in some detail in chapter 12. Tai Chi can increase the total amount of time spent sleeping while reducing the amount of time it takes to fall asleep. It also improves balance and muscle strength, both of which are important to maintain as we age, especially since one of the leading causes of hospitalization in elderly individuals is falling. Making a conscious effort to improve physical activity and exercise will support your efforts to optimize your sleep behavior, and support the other cornerstones of brain fitness as well.

Approaches To Changing Your Sleep Patterns

Several possibilities exist for adjusting your sleep patterns. These typically include two general approaches that you can use alone or in combination. The first is pharmacological (drug) therapy, which we won't cover much in this book. The second set of approaches fall into the category of behavioral therapies, which range from those you can implement on your own to those most effective if supervised by a clinical specialist.

The Red Pill Or The Blue Pill?

There are numerous over-the-counter and prescription drugs available, but unlike Neo from the movie, *The Matrix*, you can change your mind later. You should coordinate any use of these with your health care provider, since they may interact with other medications. Further, if drug intervention is necessary then you should spend some time investigating the underlying cause of your sleep disturbance, since tailoring of pharmacological treatments may more specifically address your own sleep/wakefulness issues. For example, people with depression who experience sleep/wake disturbances may benefit from changing antidepressant medications, as some antidepressant drugs cause drowsyness or increased wakefulness, which may be a desired side effect.

Behavioral

A variety of behavioral approaches are available and may be effective for individuals to implement on their own, particularly if the sleep disturbance is of a behavioral nature and not the result of another condition. If your sleep problems are due to, for example, staying up to watch television, surfing the internet, or trying to get more work done, then behavioral approaches are worth trying before moving onto the drugs.

Sleep Hygiene

The easiest approach for you to implement on your own is to attend to your sleep hygiene, although there are professionals available to help with this approach as well. The basic idea of sleep hygiene is to adhere to general guidelines about health practices and environmental factors that promote optimal sleep and avoid SOS (sub-optimal-sleep). For example, someone who is trying to improve their sleep hygiene would start to exercise regularly, not drink caffeine within five hours of their bedtime, and not eat a heavy or spicy meal just before going to bed. This person would also avoid noise when trying to go to bed (turn the radio and television off), and make sure their room is at a comfortable temperature or that they have adjusted their bedding appropriately so they aren't too hot or cold. The combination of these efforts should produce optimal sleeping opportunities. As we mentioned in the exercise and nutrition sections, the first step is to back up and assess your current condition. You may be very surprised at the habits you unconsciously engage in that make falling asleep challenging for you.

Other behavioral treatments such as sleep restriction therapy and stimulus control therapy are similar to sleep hygiene, but involve specific scheduling and use of psychological techniques to strengthen associations between sleep and the bedroom. You can try these types of techniques on your own, but they may be most effective under the supervision of a clinical specialist.

Relaxation Training

Another approach that people can try is relaxation training. Relaxation training attempts to target and reduce tensions that may inhibit our ability to fall asleep whether they are psychological or somatic. Progressive muscle relaxation is a classic example, which is an approach to address muscle tension, and can work very well for some people.

An aspect of relaxation training also addresses the psychological tension that hinders the ability to fall asleep. Meditation and imagery training are part of this general approach. We addressed these mental exercises in more detail in chapters 11 and 12, so we will briefly discuss their relevance to sleep here. Both these approaches can be exceptionally helpful in reducing the negative feelings surrounding our perception of an event, whether it has happened, or has yet to occur. Employing techniques of 'mindfulness', meditating to gain control over our emotional reactions, or envisioning your control over the positive outcome in a situation can have substantial effects on stress levels.

Other considerations we would like to put forth, from our personal experiences, are effective organization and prioritization. People who have a lot going on, or who tend to fall into the 'Type-A' personality profile tend to have problems with this, particularly if they aren't organizing effectively or if they have a tendency to take too much on (for which we raise our guilty hands). You can waste a lot of time lying awake in bed repeatedly going over schedules and tasks. The ability to entrust your scheduling to some sort of system you find dependable and works well for you can greatly reduce this type of psychological tension. And nothing snaps you out of that blissful, floating transition towards sleep like the feeling of panic elicited by your uncertainty of whether your appointment is at 8 am tomorrow or next Tuesday, and if it is next Tuesday does it conflict with the meeting you scheduled three weeks earlier.

The second, related problem can be a difficult one, prioritize. Do the tasks and responsibilities that you've taken on make sense for you and help you move towards your big-picture goal? Or are you trying to please everyone and killing yourself in the process?

Sleep Phases & Sleep Phase Shifting

Self-assessment is a critical step. Sleep is easy to neglect, and we have so many synthetic options to help us get through the day without a beneficial nap or force ourselves to fall asleep to conform to our busy schedules. However, these approaches can lead to problems that can quickly spiral out of our control. It is obvious to most of us, at least in the short-term, when we don't get enough sleep. Getting up and going the next day will be uncomfortable, and we will likely experience a lull in the mid-afternoon. But with a day or two of decent sleep, we can get back to feeling fairly normal in a relatively short amount of time. The problem is that accumulating small chunks of sleep deprivation (for example losing 1-hour a night for a month), can influence our daily function. Research is starting to show the effect of missing an hour of sleep every night, and it doesn't look that good for those of us working in the red.

During your self-assessment one thing you will want to to be aware of is when your natural sleep rhythm occurs and how long it lasts. You can begin to adjust and tinker (within reason) when you sleep, but how long you sleep allows less room for play as far is your health is concerned. The first step is to determine how long of a sleeper you are. Research shows that there are (broadly categorized) two types of sleepers: long-sleepers, and short-sleepers. Long sleepers tend to require 7.5 to 9.5 hours of sleep per night, while short-sleepers function well on 5 to 8 hours of sleep per night. Clearly, there is some overlap, but the take-home message is that you need to determine how much sleep is optimal for you. Most of us already have a good idea, even if we have been lying to ourselves for years, wanting to get by on less sleep than we actually need.

Resetting The Rhythm

There are two approaches to adjusting your bedtime in order to find your optimal sleep rhythm. You can think of these as the "pull" or "push" on your sleep times. Pulling your sleep time involves getting up at a specified time in the morning, and then eventually going to bed earlier. This is more relevant if you are having trouble falling asleep, even if you are scheduling a reasonable bedtime to go to sleep. With this approach, you will in essence "pull" your time of falling asleep down, for example from 11:30 to 10:30.

In contrast, "pushing" your sleep is a little more drastic and involves staying up later until you move your bedtime completely around the 24-hour clock in order to you find your desired time of falling asleep. To accomplish this, you need the luxury of taking a couple days off from your normal commitments (work, volunteering, etc) to allow your period of sleep to transition through times of the day that would normally require you to be up and about. You'll need time to slowly shift your sleep period around the clock. This may seem impractical and most people will find that their normal rhythm isn't drastically different from what they've been doing. However, if you are someone who is trying to force an unnatural sleep period onto your physiology, then this exercise may help.

Balance

Sleep may be an area where it would be easy to say that "more is better," particularly if you're talking with an individual between 12 and 22 years of age. As with many topics in this book, we want to promote balanced approaches to refining your lifestyle behaviors to optimize your EPIC performance.

Sleep deprivation increases risk for a number of diseases and hampers your daily function. Interestingly, too much sleep appears to affect our bodies in many of the same ways. Oversleeping increases risk for cardiovascular disease, diabetes, stroke, obesity, and cognitive impairment. So this is another case where you need to strive for balance, and will want to pay particular attention to your behavior. Something like exercise might be a little more obvious if we start doing too much, but sleep appears to have a narrow window in terms of what is 'optimal' for most people. We'll go into more detail about the U-shaped response (introduced chapter 1) to sleep in chapter 16.

This is a time when integrating a systematic approach to your sleep habits can really provide a boon to your quality of life. Work on each of the cornerstones of brain fitness will help reinforce the progress and stability of efforts made on the others. These benefits do not occur in a vacuum; they play off and support each other. But in the same turn, they can undermine and reduce your return on the effort if you neglect one area over another. So, if you're working hard to increase your mental activity, physical activity, and engage in good nutrition, but are getting lousy sleep you may undermine much of the effort you have put towards the other three cornerstones.

Moving On

We hope we've impressed upon you the idea that sleep is not wasted time and that you need to give yourself permission to sleep. In the following chapters we'll see how important and integral sleep is to our brain fitness, so don't you dare doze off.

Neural Nugget #5 – Shielding Yourself From Stress

We talked about stress in a previous neural nugget that we need to revisit as part of this discussion on allostatic load. When thinking about stress we should remember that psychological stress starts in the mind and the brain. Our perception of a situation will determine how we react to it. Whether or not a situation stresses us out or makes us 'stressy' (a term coined by Steven Colbert) will depend on how we perceive it.

Now we need stress to a point. If you're walking to your car after a long day at work and a North American Grizzly bear jumps onto the path between you and your car, you should be stressed. You need your fright, fight or flight response (we would recommend fright in this circumstance), but once you have gotten out of the situation you need to shut it off. In contrast, getting whipped into a frenzy and worrying about who will be the next American Idol for weeks on end is not really a great use of your stress response. Having your stress response turned on for extended periods of time is particularly bad.

Allostasis is our natural drive to be in balance, to turn off the stress response when we don't need it and to deal with the lifestyle choices we make. Allostatic load is the amount of effort that your brain and body must put towards allostasis (striving for balance) and depends on your genetic makeup, your exposure to stress, and the lifestyle choices you make. Good lifestyle choices and low stress coupled with a 'good genetic makeup' is the best combination. Poor genetic makeup accompanied by poor lifestyle choices and high stress is the combination you want to avoid. Many of us will fall somewhere in between but we have a lot of control over our lifestyle choices.

When you engage in healthy lifestyle choices you are helping your body more efficiently regain balance when it meets a challenge like the flu. In contrast, not avoiding poor lifestyle choices, or refusing to engage in healthy choices makes for more of an uphill battle when you have to tackle a problem like the flu, or a Grizzly bear. The effort and processes that your brain and body must make to maintain balance come at a price. They produce wear-and-tear on the brain and body. The affect of the allostatic load, the wear-and-tear, will depend on how well we are able to bring ourselves back into balance. So how do lifestyle choices help us?

We are stuck with the genes we've been given. But, as was discussed in Neural Nugget #1, A New Pair of Genes, you do have some control over those genes, and engaging in healthy lifestyle choices (e.g. not smoking) can go a long way in influencing them. In addition, managing stress is a large part of the equation.

Take our soldiers for example, in the illustration following this nugget. These guys have had to march over some rocky terrain to get to the battlefield, and now they are faced with some in-coming arrows from enemy archers. The arrows represent things that will add to the allostatic load. For example, a parent that has Alzheimer's, insulin resistance, stress at work, loss of a loved one, or the flu.

You can see that the soldier on the right probably has a better genetic makeup and may exercise a little more than our friend on the left. The soldier on the right has the benefit of good genes and looks to be healthy and in shape. It doesn't seem like the hike over the rough terrain tired him out too much. Plus he has a nice thick shield of healthy lifestyle choices that he can use to block some of the incoming arrows.

On the other hand, the soldier on the left hasn't been bestowed with the same genetic makeup. He appears to be a little tired from the hike, and is having some trouble keeping his shield in a good position to protect him from the arrows. In addition, he hasn't been taking care of his shield, so the armor that make up the shield is thin and even has some holes in it.

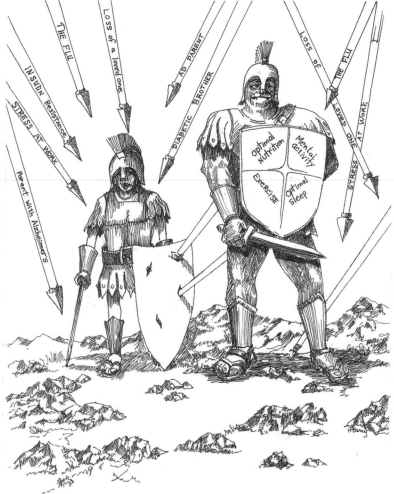

"Your ability to handle stress depends on your genes and your lifestyle choices. Since you have some control over both, which soldier would you rather be?"

Which one of these two fellows do you think is more likely to make it out of this situation under their own volition? Even if our more susceptible friend did make it out (maybe he only got an arrow in the leg or dodged them altogether) how many more volleys of archer fire will he be able to survive? Which armor would you rather wear?

So when it comes down to it, your genetic makeup can give you a leg up, or place you at a disadvantage. But the armor you choose to wear are a result of the choices that you make and can contribute substantially to the final result.

CHAPTER 15

SLEEPY FEELINGS

Sleep Ror Emotional Regulation

"The best cure for insomnia is to get a lot of sleep."
- W.C. Fields (comedian and actor)

This is a no-brainer, obvious to everyone, right? Too little sleep, we become grumpy or overly reactive to situations that would normally not trigger such a dramatic emotional response. However, we'll go beyond the obvious in this chapter to discuss how the brain responds to sleep deprivation in a very systematic way and how these systematic responses can be subtle and dangerous to your emotional intelligence and overall brain fitness.

With SOS (sub-optimal sleep) we'll start to see inappropriate emotional responses to situations that would not normally cause us to fly off the handle. This is when the grocery-store cashier really gets it on the chin because he couldn't take the expired coupon we gave him; or when we lose our temper for getting pickles on our burger when we asked for no pickles; not to mention our reduced tolerance for our fellow drivers on the road.

The point is that our ability to effectively interact in social settings is important. Throughout history, we've found there to be safety in numbers, and an overall increased effectiveness when we have social cooperation. Part of our ability to accomplish grandiose projects is the ability to dampen overly reactive emotional responses. Even constructive criticism can be tough to swallow if you've really poured your heart and soul into a project.

From a social standpoint, productivity and team building can be severely undermined if you're not at peak emotional performance. You can't have Bill punching Fred in the mouth because Fred sat in 'Bill's chair' during the staff meeting. There are likely other places to sit so it really shouldn't be an issue for Bill. If Bill insists on sitting in his favorite chair, a more tempered approach would be to ask Fred if he would be willing to move, instead of socking him in the gob. The amount of sleep Bill has been getting lately, largely determines the response he will choose to Fred's insolence.

If you're a Star Trek fan you know that no deflector shields, no photon-torpedoes, just life-support, was always the 'sitting-duck' scenario for Captain Kirk and the crew of the USS Enterprise; a situation usually paired with Romulans or Klingons bearing down on them. What we're trying to get across is that, with too much sleep deprivation, there will come a point where we are so sleep deprived that, as in the Star Trek scenario, it will take most of our brain's efforts to maintain basic life-support. This includes functions like breathing, heart rate, blood pressure, temperature regulation, and eventually, with too little sleep, even these could fail.

Clinicians have assumed for some time that mood and psychiatric disorders cause changes in sleep patterns, moving their patients into SOS. What has recently come to light is the possibility that SOS, itself, may influence or precipitate mood disorders (push you over the edge, so to speak). With that in mind, remember our <i>Neural Nugget #5, Shielding Yourself from Stress</i>. SOS puts a huge dent in the armor of our shield. It makes our metabolism, hormones and ability to learn and remember, vulnerable to the incoming arrows that contribute to your allostatic load. Developing problems in those areas can be quite unnerving, to say the least. If the load becomes too much it may push you into higher risk for developing a mood disorder. What if, on top of everything else, you experience a significant or major life event, like the death of a loved one. That, in and of itself, is a considerable obstacle, even for those who have plenty of cognitive and emotional reserve in their bank accounts. If you're already running short on sleep it can push you into a clinical mood condition. Getting enough sleep is one way to help you deal with your 'life load' and reduce your risk of developing depression.

Emotionality & Stress

During sleep, the systems in our brain and body that control our stress response have a chance to relax. Stress hormones, like norepinephrine and cortisol, decrease and the brain circuits that control our heart rate and blood pressure ramp down. SOS increases the activity of these stress-promoting systems, particularly when sleep disturbances occur over an extended period of time. Remember, that the ill effects of several nights of restricted sleep can sneak up on us, so we probably don't pay much notice until they reach a point we can no longer ignore.

There also appear to be negative physical changes in our brain and body that occur with prolonged SOS. Changes in the connections that our brain cells make and the ability to make new connections will suffer with sub-optimal-sleep. These changes can have profound effects on how we react at hormonal, emotional and cognitive levels to stress. We discussed the positive benefits of these types of changes, or 'plasticity', in chapter 13. Too much SOS is an example of how our brain's plasticity can work against us. We'll cover some of the specifics regarding the negative effects of SOS on plasticity in the next chapter.

Research demonstrates physical changes in our stress-response after several nights of restricted sleep. The kicker, or double-whammy if you will, is that these changes occur at several levels of the stress-axis. For example, the effectiveness of a hormone in the brain, called corticotrophin releasing hormone (CRH), decreases. CRH normally initiates a cascade of brain-hormone responses that ultimately lead to the release of the 'stress hormone', cortisol, from your adrenal glands. If you believe all the rants you see on late-night weight loss infomercials about the evils of cortisol, you might think that anything to reduce it, is a good thing. Well, it's not. Cortisol has several important jobs to do and appropriate control over it is required for health. However, as we've pointed out before, increasing levels of cortisol and stress for extended periods of time is when you get into trouble. But the reduction of CRH activity caused by SOS is not the end of this stressful story. Even though CRH is less effective up in our noggins, our adrenal glands become more sensitive to one of its lackeys, the hormone ACTH, which tells them to release more cortisol. This means that your control over cortisol gets very messed up when you're not sleeping well, and this is bad news for stress control and brain health.

CRH also has the ability to suppress appetite. So decreased levels after sleep deprivation may be part of the reason people with sleep loss often gain more weight; they are hungrier (remember our U-shaped curve). Couple this increased hormonal drive to eat with increased stress, which also causes many people to reach for comfort foods, and you have a recipe for packing on the pounds.

So how does this all fit in? It's safe to say that the actual mechanisms behind why these changes in stress response and emotionality occur will be somewhat complex. For example CRH, is involved in not only stress response, but also, bodyweight management, and fear and anxiety responses. However, changing the function of that protein alone doesn't fix all those disorders. Unless it is a case of extreme disease, and those cases do happen, the first step towards correcting these problems should be to assess our personal behavior and implement changes that will improve multiple aspects of our lives. Obtaining optimal sleep is one of those key behaviors.

Perception Of Stressful Events

Another issue with how sleep affects your stress response has to do with your perception of the stress. We will discuss this concept in the context of sleep effects on your cognitive ability in chapter 17, as well. In situations that you have encountered many times before, that you expect or can predict, you won't have too much of a problem perceiving correctly, even when you're tired. However, when you're thrown a curveball or a problem comes up where your standard solution doesn't work, these are the situations where the emotional deficits due to SOS become readily apparent. You don't want to view a harmless kitten as a ferocious tiger, or vice versa. In the former case, you may overact or behave completely inappropriately. In the latter case, you may get yourself into a sticky situation that you have difficulty getting out of.

Medical residents are always good for an interesting research study. They have finished medical school and are getting specific hands-on training with more experienced docs, so their stress levels are ratcheted up a couple notches. With that in mind, sleep deprivation in medical residents (which is not uncommon) has the ability to intensify the negative emotional feelings and perceptions of unexpected and disruptive events. Put another way, they don't deal well with surprises when they are tired and stressed as is the case for most people. But if you're coming into the emergency room this is definitely a situation where you want the people helping you to operate at peak performance!

In line with effects of sleep and stress on medical residents' performance, those who experience insomnia are at an increased risk for developing depression. We'll get more deeply into the interaction between SOS and depression in an upcoming section. Hopefully, you are starting to appreciate (if you didn't already) how sleep loss can result in changes in emotional performance. A minor problem that 'rocks the boat' a little suddenly becomes a major crisis. All because of how you perceive the situation.

Missed Sleep And Mood Disorders

If you've ever been fishing and attempted to use a fishing reel, particularly if you've never used one before, you will have a vivid image of a bird's nest. This is, essentially, what you get when you try to cast your line into the water and you don't know what you're doing. Once you zip the line out, the spindle ends up moving faster than the speed of the fishing line as it leaves the end of the pole and you end up with a big obnoxious tangle in your reel that more often than not (speaking from experience, or more appropriately, inexperience) is best fixed by cutting out the tangle.

This image of a bird's nest is a good analogy for the relationship between sleep disturbances and a number of mood disorders. They are often, and complexly, intertwined that it's hard to tell where one starts, the other one ends and how you would go about straightening out the line. Sleep deprivation causes changes in mood in healthy individuals and many people who have mood disorders experience very unfulfilling sleep. Like a dog chasing its tail, it's a vicious cycle.

This extra toll that sub-optimal-sleep adds to people with existing mood or cognitive disorders, is a major problem. Think back to a time when you had a few days of SOS, and how it changed your perception of events that would normally be quite benign; how much more difficult it was to integrate new information. Imagine how this must affect a person with depression, schizophrenia, or Alzheimer's disease. SOS is bad enough when you're emotional and cognitive control is working well. If those systems are already compromised, then losing sleep is quite a hit.

So What's The Worst That Can Happen?

As we discussed above, there is an intimate interaction between sleep and mood disorders. Having one will put you at risk for developing the other. This is reminiscent of the relationship we discussed between metabolic syndrome and depression in chapter 8. In fact, there are interactions between many of the topics discussed in this book, which makes a balanced approach to brain fitness through focus on all the cornerstones, so important.

<u>Losing Sleep Over Depression</u>

A person with insomnia has 4 times the risk of developing depression compared to a person without insomnia and at least one in five people diagnosed with insomnia will also have depression. The odds for someone with insomnia developing a panic disorder have been reported as 20 times higher. This doesn't mean that you will always develop a mood disorder if you have insomnia, but it speaks to the negative effect of SOS on your ability to handle the rest of the allostatic load, discussed in *Neural Nugget #5, Shielding Yourself from Stress*. Those daily stressors we encounter, the unexpected, sometimes traumatic life events that can catch us when we are least aware, all test our capacity to carry more load. If these are piled on top of the stress of poor sleep (and potentially poor diet, lack of exercise, lack of active stress management) then they can precipitate very serious physical and mental health problems. Optimal sleep will help protect the emotional and cognitive bank account we have worked so hard to achieve.

Depression imposes a major psychological, physical, emotional and financial burden on the people afflicted with the disorder, those that are close to them, and society as a whole. Approximately 1 out of 5 people will experience serious depression at some point in their life, and the risk increases as you age.

Is there a way to reduce your risk of developing depression? Yes. Although there are genetic components to depression, most of your risk is defined by the combination of genetic factors and what we experience in our environment. Going back to the allostatic load concept, if you have a good genetic makeup you may be able to carry extra armor that will protect you from the onslaught of allostatic overload. If you are like the smaller soldier, you won't be able to carry the extra armor and therefore won't be able to handle as heavy of an allostatic onslaught. One of the best things you can do for yourself is to strive to live in a way that will reduce the likelihood that you will develop a mood disorder and getting optimal sleep is a huge factor in that. Disrupted sleep patterns occur so frequently in certain mood disorders, that they are part of the criteria for diagnosing the disorder. In fact, only 1 percent of depressed patients don't have insomnia. This again, illustrates the strength of the association between SOS and mood disorders.

Unfortunately, insomnia is particularly problematic for older individuals. More than half of the risk of depression in elderly community-dwelling individuals is attributed to insomnia, second only to major bereavement (e.g. loss of a loved one). As we get older our sleep starts to change, which is why this is such an important area to stay aware of and ready to protect; and why we spend so much time drilling this point into your brain in this chapter.

Working sooner, rather than later to optimize sleep can provide huge boost even to people that already have depression. When followed over time, people with depression and unresolved insomnia are almost 40 times as likely to become depressed again within a year's time, compared to people who were able to resolve their sleep problems. So, if you or someone you care about suffers from depression, working towards optimal-sleep will help decrease the likelihood of cycling back into a depressed state. Listening to those late night sleeping pill commercials is not the best approach, either. If you truly have a problem sleeping you should consider seeing a sleep professional who will work with you to figure out why you are not sleeping. Even if you don't currently suffer from mood problems, if you have disrupted sleep the time to start working to improve is now.

The importance of attending to sleep problems early is highlighted by a 30-year study that followed a group 1,053 young men, who were medical students at the study's onset. Researchers looked at their sleep habits in medical school and followed them for several decades. Over the course of the study, the effects of lack of sleep began to unveil something intriguing. The men that reported insomnia during medical school were twice as likely to develop depression over the next few years. Importantly, none of the participants included in the study had depression before they graduated from medical school.

This study cannot draw the conclusion that sleep loss in that isolated time-frame (medical school) had the ability to cause depression later down the road, but it impressively predicted the increased risk of depression. Of course, other factors may all be related, such as coping strategies that helped protect some of the physicians, while others were more vulnerable to the cumulative load of stress and SOS. However, the link between early sleep problems and later depression seems to continue to rear its ugly head, reaffirming the importance of not letting your SOS get out of control.

Anxious For Sleep

Anxiety disorders are, unfortunately, another common problem. In the United States estimates are that 25 percent of people are experiencing anxiety problems. Studies that look at large numbers of people have indicated that the onset of anxiety disorders closely precedes the onset of a variety of sleep problems. In a large survey of people in European countries, approximately 25% of those surveyed had an anxiety disorder, similar to that found in the US. Additionally, 40% of people with an anxiety disorder experienced insomnia at the onset of their problems, while another 34% experienced insomnia after developing the disorder. This is important because the link between depression and insomnia follows a different time-course. Where insomnia seems to start before or at the same time as a depressive disorder, it seems to start with or follow development of anxiety problems. Due to the large comorbidity of sleep and anxiety disorders, scientists believe that a substantial portion of the insomnia problem in the general public is associated with, or caused by, an anxiety disorder.

So, it's probably pretty clear that this is another situation where things could easily spiral out of control. As you become anxious about a given situation, your preoccupation with it may result in greater difficulty falling asleep. As you begin to become sleep deprived, you may become anxious about the fact that you're not sleeping well and how this will impact your performance during regular waking hours. In addition, the lack of optimal sleep may, in and of itself, produce subtle changes in how you perceive and react to other stressors and increase your odds for depression.

We are trying to raise your awareness to realize this is happening so you can make a deliberate effort to correct it. You also need to remember that you do not need to face this on your own. Family, friends, support groups and clinical professionals are available to help you reorient yourself. Strong social support networks are invaluable, whether working through a very serious problem like an anxiety disorder, or simply trying to make vegetables a part of your normal routine. Keep your connections strong!

Wreaking Havoc On Our Emotions

Why does sleep loss cause so many problems? Sleep is a time to recharge our batteries, and this is very true in terms of brain regions that regulate your behavioral arousal. Your frontal cortex serves as the brake for other brain regions that control your emotional response to social and environmental situations. It's the well behaved part of the brain that stops you from telling your boss he or she is an idiot, from telling the guy next to you on the bus he really needs a shower, or composing a flaming response to a co-workers thoughtless email, and actually sending it. Sleep has the ability to restore and promote optimal function of your frontal cortex and the animalistic regions that it controls. But, when we are sleep deprived, our social etiquette brakes begin to fail and our primitive self comes out. It's like Dr. Jekyll losing control to Mr. Hyde. Interestingly, the frontal cortex does not fully develop until the age of 18 to 22, which may explain some things in your house.

Recognizing social cues and appropriately responding to situations are high-level functions, particularly if you consider that we humans do much of this with language. These are very important skills to have and use correctly. Think about how awkward a situation can feel when someone's response to a tragic event is laughter. The mood of the room and the social dynamic will change very quickly. Many times changes in the social context aren't so blatant, but they do occur. Think about how you've felt when you've asked for help or feedback in a group setting and response has been sarcastic or scolding.

Some of these skills can have subtle effects on our 'survival' and it takes some foresight to predict what the consequences of our actions will be. We need to know that blowing off the bosses email to update the client database will not work in our favor when our time for promotion comes up. However, we would likely survive a poor decision here, even if it meant lower pay or a different job. Yet, most of the time we want more than simple survival. For this, we need the ability to get through the line at the grocery store without snapping at the cashier. We need the ability to act compassionately towards someone who is an hour late to a scheduled meeting. Those are the skills that suffer with SOS, and require much more effort and awareness to bring them back.

Loss of these skills can threaten our survival when our ability to drive a car suffers with sleep deprivation. We've already mentioned that sleep deprivation results in performance indistinguishable to that of someone who has had several alcoholic drinks. But the car is very often a place where many people not only feel safe, in control, but empowered. Almost invincible. Combine SOS with an undeveloped frontal cortex of a teenager driver and you have the reason why their insurance rates are so high.

If our SOS gets bad enough, our brains begin to completely redirect the priority from the higher set of social functions to those most critical for life. This is where we experience the star-trek scenario, *Wrath of Khan*, as it were. No

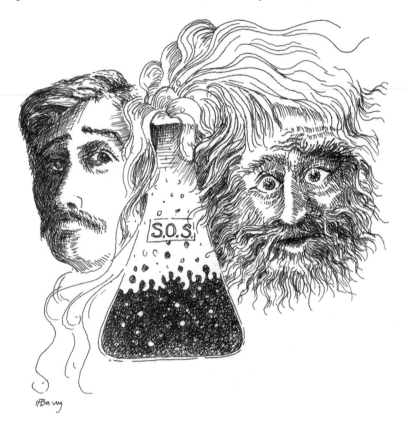

Emotional regulation suffers when we are tired. SOS can transition you into Mr. Hyde. Luckily, optimal sleep is the antidote that can bring you back."

photon torpedoes, the transporter room is off-line and the shields are down. All we have is that red mood lighting on the bridge and Spock calmly telling us that the human reaction to such a situation is "peculiar."

Moving On

Remember, now is the time to save up, to grow your reserves so we have the physical, cognitive and emotional bank account to better handle unexpected problems. In the next section, we'll explore how SOS alters the physical nature of our bodies and brains. SOS can cause maladaptive changes to the anatomy of your brain, but will it really impact our efforts on the other three cornerstones of brain fitness?

Let's find out.

CHAPTER 16

SLEEP! IT DOES A BRAIN GOOD
Sleeping For Physical Intelligence

"That we are not much sicker and much madder than we are is due exclusively to that most blessed and blessing of all natural graces, sleep."

- Aldous Huxley (writer and humanist)

Science has started to recognize the profound impact that sleep has on our health. This recognition has taken place in just the past 10 to 15 years. For a long time the main symptom of sleep deprivation that concerned people was daytime sleepiness. Pesky yes, but hardly a major public health issue. Daytime sleepiness was more of a concern for managers who wanted to optimize productivity at work, not for family physicians trying to keep you vibrant and healthy. As research continues to accumulate, however, it appears that sub-optimal-sleep (SOS) goes well beyond causing a little tiredness, to increasing the risk for a number of health problems affecting our cardiovascular, hormone, immune, and nervous systems, not to mention potential occupational hazards. In this chapter, we'll discuss how sleep loss affects not only our mood and cognition, but our metabolic function as well. These effects can translate into obesity, diabetes, and heart disease. We'll show you more reasons why living *BrainFit* will help keep your body fit as well.

Weight & Metabolism

A U-shaped curve is a good way to describe the interaction between sleep and measures of obesity. We talked about the inverse-U shaped curve in this book's introduction and in the previous sections to illustrate the idea that more is only better to a point, after which more can become detrimental. The U-shaped curve is a great example of why we should pay attention to how we live and strive to maintain balance. As we've discussed many times before, the need for balance holds true in several aspects of our mind and body so it is important to be on the lookout for them. So too is it with sleep. With too little sleep, body weight tends to increase. With too much of it, body weight also goes up. But there's a sweet-spot in the middle, an optimal amount of sleep that is not associated with weight gain. That's where we want to be.

In chapter 14, we mentioned sleep loss trends over the last few decades and how they correlate with the increase in obesity rates. To reiterate, the percentage of men and women who sleep less than 6 hours per night has increased between 7 and 15% over the past 35 years. That's a big chunk of people (no pun intended) who are getting far less sleep than we used to. As we've pointed out before, it's a disturbing coincidence that these decreases in sleep behavior have paralleled the increased rates of obesity in the United States. For sure, sleep is not the only factor in the plumping of our society, but the emerging data sure make it seem like it's an important one.

Hormone Systems

Sleep regulates the rhythm of many hormone systems in your brain and body. Some hormones are high when you're asleep and low when you're awake. Others are low when you sleep and high when you're up and about. These cycles of hormones, which are all part of your circadian rhythm, are an important part of keeping your physiology on track. SOS can derail this process and wreak havoc on several systems. We'll discuss some of the important ones here.

We've talked a lot about exercise, and have mentioned how exercise can improve sleep quality. But these two aspects of our lives go hand in hand. Sleep is an essential part of the recovery process from exercise. It is a time that our bodies use to build up and restore our muscles. Bodybuilders are people who really know how to exploit this system. Hormones that build muscle increase during sleep. Very serious bodybuilders will lift weights, eat, and then sleep two to three times during the day. Sounds kind of nice doesn't it? Lift, eat, sleep, and repeat. Well, at least the eating and sleeping part sounds good.

SOS also causes changes in the level of hormones that tell your brain you're hungry or that you don't really need to eat right now. Leptin is a hormone that tells your brain you have plenty of energy stored in your body and informs your brain that we don't need any more food. Your levels of leptin decrease after sleep deprivation, which takes the brakes off the eating process, since you won't get the appropriate 'stop eating' signal. This is one reason why SOS associates with weight gain. Further leptin plays a role in controlling mood and cognition. So messing with your emotional system, while simultaneously messing with your eating drive, can have far-reaching effects. We all know that mood and food go hand in hand and you don't want to lose control of the hormones that regulate this. To double the whammy, sleep deprivation also increases levels of a hormone called ghrelin. In some ways, ghrelin has actions opposite to leptin. It is a hormone released by your stomach to tell your brain that your stomach is empty and you should eat. So SOS decreases leptin, a hormone telling you to stop eating; and increases ghrelin, a hormone telling you you're hungry.

Another important pair of weight controlling hormones regulated by sleep are growth hormone and thyroid stimulating hormone. Growth hormone plays many roles in driving energy away from fat storage and toward building strong muscles and bones. Thyroid stimulating hormone activates our thyroid and profoundly influences how we burn calories at rest. So this pair has a lot to do with storage and burning of calories. With total sleep deprivation, our growth hormone levels plummet, and return to normal only after a period of rebound sleep. However, in chronic partial sleep loss, growth hormone does not normalize. With SOS-induced low growth hormone levels, you will develop a tendency to store more energy in fat cells and less in muscle over time. In addition, levels of thyroid stimulating hormone substantially drop after 3-5 days of partial sleep deprivation. This adds to a decrease in the calories you'll burn at rest. The last paragraph detailed how sleep loss can drive you to eat more. Now we're telling you that SOS also causes you to use those extra calories to make more fat and burn less when you're resting. We'd like to point out the ramifications of this. If you are frustrated with how long it takes for an exercise program to help you reasonably lose weight (several weeks), think about how much longer it will take if you have SOS. You may be undoing much of your hard work at the gym.

To sum up the issue of sleep deprivation regarding hormone systems that affect energy metabolism (and these are just a few of many hormone disturbances), we have some major problems. First, your drive to eat will increase while you will have less brake activity to tell you to stop eating. Second, your drive to store fat will increase while your drive to build muscle and bone will decrease. Third, your drive to burn calories will decrease. It's not too much of a stretch then, to say you will dramatically boost your odds of gaining weight, which puts you at increased risk for diabetes and cardiovascular disease. All because of a little less shut eye. WOW!

Burning Calories While You Sleep

We just mentioned burning calories while you're at rest, which may have raised your eyebrow. But we do burn a lot of calories at rest, especially during sleep. You may think of sleep as a very inactive time from an energy burning perspective. It's seems a time when you are in a state of hibernation or suspended animation. You'd expect all your bodily functions to slow to a crawl and your energy expenditure to drop to practically zero. Kind of like those pods they used in the movie, *Aliens*, for extended space travel.

In contrast to our little sci-fi fantasy of hibernation, you actually burn a fair amount of calories as you sleep. In fact, you are always burning some calories no matter what we're doing throughout the day. When you are at rest (lying quietly), the amount of calories that you burn is referred to as your basal metabolic rate. A variety of things can influence your basal metabolic rate including your ratio of muscle to fat. Since muscle is more metabolically active than fat, the higher your muscle to fat ratio, the higher your basal metabolic rate and the more calories you burn just lying around. Now if our hibernation idea held true you'd be stuck at the basal metabolic rate for the duration of your nightly sleep, but that's not what happens.

When we sleep, we actually go through several different levels of energy expenditure. We already talked about the stages of sleep in chapter 14, now we'll give you an insight into how that impacts your calorie burning. For example, during non-REM sleep you tend to burn fewer calories compared to REM sleep. If you remember from previous sections, non-REM sleep is more common during the first half of the night and you have proportionally more REM sleep in the second half of the night. As you begin to cycle through REM sleep your levels of energy utilization increase. Said another way, when you are in the very active portion of sleep (REM sleep), which is when you dream and are easily awakened, you are burning more calories. Maybe running away from that boogie monster is more real than you think (although our ability to move our muscles is suppressed during REM sleep, probably to protect us from acting out our dreams).

This is important for several reasons. When we become sleep-deprived we lose time from our REM sleep since we need to cycle through non-REM sleep before we can enter REM sleep. So what becomes a big problem is that when we have self-imposed (behavioral) sleep-deprivation or disrupted sleep, we will be cheated out of our REM sleep. By losing sleep we are actually cheating ourselves out of burning calories at a higher rate, particularly if we are experiencing reduced REM sleep. Those are calories we can burn that we don't even need to be awake for! A week of solid sleep sounds better than an extra 20 minutes twice a week on the stair master.

Take Dave for example. Dave has disrupted sleep and wakes up an average of four times per night. Each time he wakes, it takes him about 20 minutes to fall back asleep. So he's already lost 1-hour and 20-minutes from his sleep time. Since it takes the average person about 90 minutes to cycle into REM sleep, in the eight-hour window that Dave has available to sleep, he's only asleep for 6-hours and 40-minutes, and could be spending as little as 40 minutes in REM sleep (if he was being awakened during REM sleep). Granted this is a very simplified and somewhat opportunistic example (everyone's math will be different), but it should help illustrate the point that sleep is important and should be protected. In experiencing

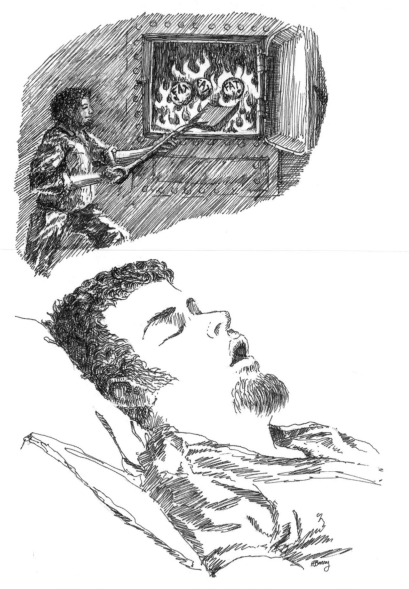

"You burn energy to help limit fat stores while you sleep. Be sure to give yourself permission to sleep so you can maintain an optimal metabolism."

this type of sleep behavior Dave has the potential to gain about 3 pounds per year (assuming it will all be fat) as a result of cheating himself out of optimal-sleep. This doesn't sound too bad, but remember that excess weight is a risk-factor for poor sleep quality. Plus, this is three pounds gained if everything else stays the same, particularly if you aren't eating excess calories. So if your exercise, eating and sleep habits aren't all that good, the pounds start to pack on quickly. We're sure you looked back on at least a couple occasions and wondered how the last several months flew by so quickly. During that time, what kind of commitment did you make to optimal sleep, how far have you let yourself slide down the spiral? As we discuss in this chapter, SOS adversely affects your insulin and glucose regulation in addition to giving you extra opportunities to eat, all of which can propel you further down the spiral. So remember that sleep isn't just good for your mood and memory it has the added benefits of burning off some extra calories during our dreamtime lumberjacking escapades.

Sleep Loss Increases The Risk For Diabetes

Early on, much of sleep-research focused on total sleep deprivation. That is to say no sleep at all during the night. Now researchers recognize that vast majority of people get some sleep each night, but probably not the full amount that they really need. Roughly defined, *chronic sleep curtailment* is the loss of one to two hours of sleep each night, below a person's amount of optimal-sleep, for an extended period of time. The impact of chronic sleep curtailment wasn't really recognized until about 15 years ago when it was linked with a number of other diseases.

As mentioned in the introductory chapter for this section, our bodies are very protective of our sleep. Your brain will attempt to force you to make up for a lost night of sleep, the following night. But our brains don't pick up so easily on our shenanigans if we just shave an hour or two per night. We can typically get through small periods of daytime drowsiness with any number of caffeinated or sugary aids, so this behavior is temporarily sustainable; not healthy, but sustainable, for a while. The effects of chronic sleep curtailment are subtle at the onset and only become obvious after an extended period, which can be months to years or even decades. This is particularly true with the effect of SOS on obesity and diabetes. Although changes in hormone systems discussed above occur after a few nights of SOS, the cumulative load resulting in outwardly recognizable changes takes longer. This means that you may not notice all the hormonal problems until they've become rather serious.

One thing we can't ignore is the impact of SOS on the regulation of blood sugar which has major implications for diabetes. Our ability to effectively use our blood sugar is lower during slow-wave sleep and higher during REM and light non-REM sleep. So experiencing SOS and losing time from our REM sleep decreases the amount of time we use our blood sugar more effectively. The more time we spend inefficiently controlling our blood sugar, the closer we get to a diabetic state. So sleep loss can push us into a pre-diabetic state and increase our odds for developing the full blown disease. Not cool. Not cool at all.

The effects of SOS in terms of blood-sugar control are really quite striking. Two nights of sleep restriction increases morning blood sugar levels and lowers insulin levels (a major hormone that controls blood sugar). So after only two nights of reduced sleep (4 hours per night), healthy individuals appeared to be insulin resistant, which is one step toward diabetes. This is an opportunity for caffeinated digression!

Hair Of The Dog

Think of what you're doing to yourself when you are already sleep deprived and then start off your day with coffee. We are definitely not coffee abstainers. The words you are reading right now were likely written next to a cup full of a nice dark roasted java. But there are clearly effects of coffee on blood-sugar physiology that are less than optimal. Coffee temporarily increases blood sugar levels by decreasing your sensitivity to insulin (as an aside, this means the worst foods to combine with coffee are sweet foods, like cookies and donuts – resulting in Clancy Wiggum instead of RoboCop). So, based on what we said above, if you're sleep deprived by a couple hours, your blood-sugar and insulin levels will be up in the morning, when you're already a little insulin resistant. To cope with our lack of sleep, what do we do? Have a cup of coffee.

Now it's not necessarily the coffee that's bad, it's how we use it, to overcome a sleep deficit. So how could you work around this issue? Obviously, the best way would be to get a full night's sleep. If your sleep wasn't the best, however, and you're in a pinch, here are a couple other options. First, you could go for a 20-30 minute walk once you wake up, while your coffee is brewing. Why? Well, exercise reduces blood sugar levels, so will help offset the temporary insulin resistance we're about to induce with our coffee. Furthermore, exercise increases vigilance and attention, so may reduce the amount of coffee we need to drink to feel awake. Alternatively, you could just give up your morning coffee all together.

Don't like that approach? Here's another option. Why not eat first and wait an hour or two before having that first cup of coffee. Why? Once you "prime the pump," so to speak, with food the effects of coffee on elevating blood glucose and insulin are less profound. Plus, delaying that first cup of coffee gives your metabolism a little more time to reset itself and bring your blood sugar back under control. As with many of the topics we've discussed in this book, timing is everything.

Bringing It Back To The Brain

So if this is a book about brain health, why are we spending so much time talking about the effects of sleep deprivation on insulin and hormones and weight gain? Well, these things all interact, and can have a profound impact on your brain's ability to function optimally. Remember your brain and body are linked....by your neck. But seriously, they are linked by much more than that. Numerous biological systems exist so that the body can tell the brain what is going on below the chin, and in turn, the brain can then help orchestrate an effective response from the body. So it's time we finally introduce them to each other. "Brain this is body, body this is brain. We hope you two will be able to work amicably together, as you'll be stuck together for life."

Sleep Deprivation And Plasticity

One of the more brain-based responses to SOS we want to discuss is the issue of plasticity or the ability of the brain to rewire itself. This is an important skill for your brain to have. You'll need it to continue to learn, adapt to, and successfully conquer the challenges that life throws at you. We've talked about this in several contexts already and will revisit it again in the next chapter. We briefly bring up plasticity here because sleep deprivation decreases the brain's ability to strengthen connections between brain cells. This, in turn, results in reduced learning. You'll remember our friend, BDNF, one of our brain's favorite fertilizers. One way that sleep deprivation may cause reduced learning capacity is through decreasing levels of BDNF in the brain. We've mentioned how exercise and challenging and diverse environments can increase BDNF. Well SOS will work against this positive benefit.

Other hormone changes caused by sleep deprivation also directly affect our ability to learn and strengthen connections between brain cells. Some may even cause brain cells to die, if they are out of whack for too long. Leptin, for example, contributes to learning and regulates mood. We already discussed how loss of sleep decreases leptin levels and contributes to weight gain. In addition, leptin is important for plasticity in the hippocampus, a brain area critical for learning and memory. With lower leptin, plasticity may be compromised and learning efficiency reduced. Furthermore, lower leptin levels can contribute to depression, which can feed back to cause problems for cognition and metabolism.

Cortisol, is another hormone we've previously discussed as influencing a lot of things in your body, and has profoundly negative effects on your brain if it remains elevated for too long. Who killed that brain cell? Was it Mrs. Cortisol, in the dining room with the candlestick? Maybe, it's hard to pin the rap totally on cortisol, but it appears that elevated cortisol along with a number of other factors tend to result in a 'sick' brain cell. Once at that point, the brain cell just needs a little hip-check to send it into the grave, which can happen with any number of stressors that normally wouldn't be devastating. Again, it all goes back to the concepts of reserve and allostatic load and sleep is crucial.

Sleep And Immune Function

The final serious concern we'll discuss in this chapter is that of your body's defense system against invading germs and viruses. Sleep deprivation adversely influences your immune system. Following sleep deprivation the body's ability to produce antibodies is reduced. Therefore, sleep deprivation dampens your immediate response to pathogens, germs and viruses. That's pretty bad if we can't mount a full defense against an outside pathogen invasion, but it gets worse. Inflammatory chemicals in the body become elevated when we are sleep deprived. Any parent will remember that sleep deprivation period that they were not ready for after the birth of their first baby. They'll remember never having felt so tired, or being sick so frequently. Again, we'd like to point out how many of these things can overlap, add to, and complicate each other. Chronically elevated stress has the ability to compromise immune system function, and sub-optimal-sleep can muck it up even further. Combine these with the effects of diet and exercise on our physical intelligence that we've already discussed, and you realize how much control you have, for better or for worse. So, now that we've chased our tails for a while, we should step back and take stock of all the facets of our lives, since they have the ability to influence each other. Maybe you should just sleep on it for a while.

Moving On

You're probably not surprised that sleep is important, but hopefully we've made you more aware of the toll that SOS takes on our bodies and brains. It actually changes our anatomy and the structure of our brain. That's great, but we have a few billion brain cells anyway. Does SOS have any influence on our ability to learn, remember, and integrate complex and abstract ideas? By now you've probably guessed that it will, so let's take a look at some methods on how to get the most memory boosting power out of our sleep.

CHAPTER 17

CLEAR AWAKENINGS

Sleeping For Cognitive Performance

"I love sleep. My life has the tendency to fall apart when I'm awake, you know?"

- Ernest Hemingway (author and journalist)

The last few chapters have highlighted the role that sleep plays in regulating your emotional and physical intelligence. The final piece in the brain fitness formula details how sleep controls your cognitive intelligence. It's no surprise that sleep, learning and memory and general cognitive abilities are tightly related. If you're tired it's difficult to absorb and process new information, let alone recall it later. But you may not realize the intricacy of the relationship between sleep and cognitive performance. Many people are especially surprised to learn that sleeping after learning is just as important of getting good rest before hand.

Priming Memory

We need to say at the outset that the field of sleep and memory is a burgeoning area of research with many exciting and interesting findings. It is also deepening in complexity as studies continue to pile up. However, we'll feed you the less controversial conclusions and stick to the goal of delivering what it means for your own EPIC performance. There are currently debates raging about which phase of sleep is important for specific processes involved in forming and recalling specific types of memory.

It is safe, however, to make the general statement that learning and remembering are intimately intertwined with sleep. But it's not just about being tired when you are trying to learn something. Memory and the more inclusive idea of 'cognition', are dependent upon our sleep before we learn, our sleep after we learn, and our sleep surrounding those times when we would like to remember what we have learned. So unless you have week-long stretches where you don't need to recall information that you have learned, you should probably make optimal-sleep a daily priority.

If you want to truly learn something and store it in long-term memory to recall it and use it later you must pay attention to your sleep habits. This is why 'cramming' is almost always a bad idea. First, most people experience some level of stress if they have left a substantial portion of their work or studies to the last minute, which in and of itself can interfere with learning. Second, as is the case with most 'traditional' cram sessions, people tend to stay up late, sacrificing sleep in an attempt to learn as much of the material as they can in a short amount of time.

Now cramming does work for some people, much to the annoyance of the rest of us. However, it is a bad strategy since overall ability to retain the material for long periods of time will suffer. Further, if your discipline which requires sequential and progressive learning, as most disciplines do, you will have to repeat this process with more effort each time you move on to the next step in your training process. You will have to fill in the holes of what you have forgotten from the last cram-session.

Storing Memory

The process of moving newly learned information to long-term storage (also known as consolidation, or the transfer of short-term to long-term memory) is well known to be affected by insufficient sleep. Scientists still debate (with some fury) the exact biological mechanisms and stages of sleep involved for the transfer of different types of memory. But those details are beyond the scope of this book because they aren't really important for what you need to do to optimize our sleep. You don't really care exactly when your memories are built. You just need to consolidate those memories efficiently and effectively.

Sleep and memory are both complex things. Researchers initially believed that memory consolidation was a distinct and short-term process. We thought that the movement of a memory from short to long-term storage happened all at once. It is now apparent, however, that this process happens in stages and can take from hours to years. So learning really is a life-long process.

What is important for our discussion on sleep is that some of the processes that transfer memories into our long-term storage occur exclusively when we are sleeping and are most efficient when we are maintaining levels of optimal-sleep. What many people don't realize is that the sleep you get after you learn something is the time when you really drive it home. This applies to both visual and motor learning as well as facts and figures. Learning covers all kinds of practical stuff like recognizing patterns or new motor skills; for finding your way around, the finer strategies of bridge or chess, or how to cast a fishing line without producing a birds nest each time. Maximizing your optimal sleep will greatly support your efforts on all these fronts.

Getting On Stage

If you'll remember (see you're already having recall what you've learned from other sections of the book) we discussed how sleep is a progressive process. It builds and changes as we repeat our sleep cycle throughout the night. The proportion of time you spend in each stage of sleep changes slightly with each subsequent cycle. Although you can't directly control the proportion of time you spend in each stage over a night of sleep, you can make sure that you get enough of your optimal-sleep time. Since sleep is progressive and continuously builds on itself throughout the night, you will miss your ability to build a full night's sleep if you don't commit to getting to bed at a reasonable hour. Likewise, if you are waking up early, for whatever reason, you're being short-changed of building in your full sleep pattern. As we discussed in earlier chapters, you get more REM sleep in each sleep cycle as you move through the night, so by the second half of the night the proportion of time you spend in REM sleep increases dramatically. What this means is that four hours is not half as good as eight hours. Since it's not a linear process, it doesn't work that way. Sleeping for four hours may only get you one-quarter of your REM sleep, as compared to the full eight. If you don't get your full sleep time, you take a substantial hit in your later stages.

But there's even more to it than that. Non-REM sleep relates more to the consolidation of motor skill tasks. While slow-wave-sleep (stages 3&4) and REM sleep seem more important for the consolidation of visual skill memory. REM sleep also appears to be important for emotional memories. There is still a lot of debate about which phase of sleep is critical for specific types of learning, but for your purposes, you only need to know that optimizing your sleep is a necessary priority for strengthening your ability to learn and remember. If you are having problems with a specific type of memory then you might do well to investigate your sleep quality with the help of a sleep professional. In this case, you'll

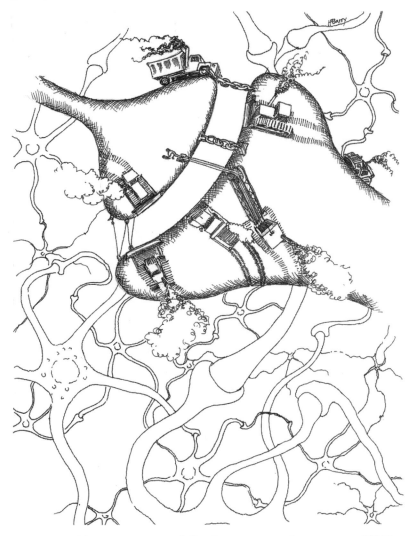

"Sleep is essential for learning and memory. While you sleep, your brain works to strengthen and stabilize synaptic connections that enhance memories of your experiences from the previous day."

want to figure out exactly which stage of sleep may be messed up, using a lot of fancy equipment and some researchers to help you out. It may be that some assistive equipment to help you sleep could do wonders. Sleep apnea (pauses in breathing during sleep) can have a substantial influence on your health and quality of life, but there are ways to address the problem. CPAP (Continuous Positive Airway Pressure) machines can help immensely, so if you think you have more than a behaviorally based sleep problem seek professional help. We've added some information in the resource section that can get you started.

Recalling Memory

A good night's sleep also greatly enhances recall of things you have already learned. Recalling memories is like placing a phone call to your brain to find out what you need to know. If you've just hung up then you can quickly reconnect by using the redial button. That works fine until you make another phone call. Then redialing the last phone number won't work because it's not the one you wanted. Sleep is like having a good pen and notepad next to the phone to write down each person's name and phone number so you can remake whichever connection when needed. If you've ever tried to write down a number with a pen that's running out of ink, you'll know how frustrating that can be. You have to turn the notepad at an angle to the light so you can try and make out the indentation created by the tip of the pen. Sleep helps you keep the pen full of ink. That way, if you get a couple more phone calls (memories) you have the ability to dial back the specific person you need to speak with.

This applies both to things that you have to recall while you are learning (immediate recall) and to the memories that you need to recall the next day where a good pen would be very handy to have. The ability to effectively recall memories is related to things called sleep-spindles, which can be seen as funny little squiggles when the brain's electrical activity is measured using an EEG (electroencephalogram). The number of sleep-spindles increases the night after we learn something new, and your ability to recall information while you are learning appears related to the number of sleep-spindles you had the previous night. In fact, researchers can record brain cells firing in a rat while the rat is learning a task; and then watch those same neurons fire in the same sequence when the rat is sleeping. The brain 'replays' the learning experience during sleep.

Think about all that hard work you do concentrating, organizing, studying, and integrating information when learning something new. If you haven't slept well the night before, it will take more effort to learn the same material. We're not saying that you couldn't learn it, but it may be more difficult. In addition, if you don't sleep well the night after you've learned something new, chances are that some of the information you worked so hard to acquire will slip away, or will be difficult to recall when you need it. This memory consolidation effect of sleep can go on for several weeks after the time we learned the new information.

In an interesting study, researchers taught participants a task and then divided them into two groups. One group was deprived of sleep the night after learning and the other group slept normally. Researchers then gave all participants three nights of good sleep before testing them on the task, so they would all be fully rested during the test. The group that slept well after learning the task, significantly out-performed the other group, even though several days had passed since the sleep deprivation.

Emotional Learning

Many things come into play when you learn something. Your emotional state (happy, sad, scared, angry) surrounding the learning event is one major factor that can influence how you learn and remember an experience. Your level of behavioral arousal also affects your ability to recognize and focus on significant events and details. So it's not surprising then that situations with a high 'emotional value' become very strong memories. We discussed this briefly in chapter 13 on the topic of adding emotional value to mental activities in order to improve learning and retention. The interaction between mood and memory is a two-way street. It can be very good, like remembering the birth of a child. Or it can be very detrimental as in negative traumatic experiences. Since we've already discussed how sleep plays a huge role in emotional regulation, you can see how sleep affects learning on multiple fronts.

The Executives Secret To Success

In previous chapters we discussed how SOS causes the brain to shut down more 'frivolous' or 'human' functions in order to conserve our more basic survival mechanisms. Many of the skills that humans have developed project so far past survival that they are considered to be 'executive' or front-office functions. These are functions like planning your shopping list, restraining your frustration when the store is out of bananas, and all kinds of other human functions. The superior complexity and development of the frontal cortex in the human brain is the home for many of these executive functions. Executive skills and the function of the frontal cortex are some of the first things to suffer from SOS. These loss of function effects are progressive, so the longer or more sleep deprived you become the more impaired your ability to problem solve and integrate new information.

Let's explore this idea with an example that should be familiar to you. Let's say that due to construction on Interstate-94, you've been taking route-121 as an alternate way to get home. On your way home at the end of a long day, just before you are about to take the 121 exit, you hear on the radio that route-121 is closed from Van Ness to Charleston Street. The detour could add an hour to your commute. If you've been getting enough sleep you may be able to make the split second decision not to take the route 121 exit, realizing you can get around this problem. You just take 94 past the closure and meet up with 121 at Riverside Drive. If you are a little sleep deprived you might just stay on auto-pilot, take the route 121 exit and now you're stuck. You have to deal with the traffic. Have you been getting enough sleep to enable this quick thinking decision and remap your route home before you get stuck in traffic that has cued up behind the closure? This is a situation where sleep deprivation can turn an easy 25-minute commute home into a 2.5-hour nightmare. How many times do you take the long way through your daily tasks because SOS has you off your game?

Failure or decreased performance of your higher-order, or executive brain function is probably the stage of sleep deprivation that everyone has experienced at some point in their life. This is when you can see the face, but can't quite remember the name of that important client. It's when you're having trouble putting together a solid plan for the order of your errands so you're not doubling back on your route. When you have trouble with executive tasks, you may still function quite normally for a short period of time, as long as you're not faced with a major challenge. You know you are a little off and that you can perform better, but these deficits aren't yet obvious to others. Only you and those close to you are probably aware that you are a little off kilter on that particular day. But what happens if this continues?

Attention And Vigilance

Your ability to pay attention to important details is an obvious requirement for your ability to learn. Consider this scenario. You've just moved to a new city. Your spouse has been there for a couple weeks finalizing the purchase of your new home. Due to obligations at your old job, you needed to transition from that job to your new job without any time off. After flying in on the red-eye you picked up your rental car and went directly to the office. You met your spouse for dinner at the end of the day near where you work and are now following him or her back to your new house.

You're tired. It's the end of a full day at a new job, after taking the red-eye that morning, but you would greatly benefit from learning a little bit about your new surroundings so you can get to work more easily the following morning. You need to learn what landmarks help you navigate from work to your new home, so you need to pay attention to where you are when you're driving. It won't do you any good to focus solely on the radio or on the back of your spouse's car. This may serve to reaffirm your knowledge of his or her political leanings and love of Star Wars after repeatedly reading the bumper stickers plastered across the back of the car, but you wouldn't have any sense of how you got back to the house. It also wouldn't be that safe to place too much of your focus on identifying new landmarks, if you do that at the expense of paying attention to other drivers or traffic signals.

Your ability to learn is heavily influenced by your ability to maintain focus and vigilance. The trick is to focus on what is relevant and important in the moment, but at the same time be aware of other aspects of the environment that you would do well to notice. The quality of your sleep affects your ability to use and balance these attention skills. As we mentioned above, activity in the prefrontal cortex of the brain, an area that is crucial for putting the brakes on situation-inappropriate behavior, is an early target that suffers from SOS. If this brain region is not functioning at its best, you'll have difficulty dividing your attention between all the things you should be keeping tabs on. You may also remember that the prefrontal cortex plays a strong role in regulating emotional responses to environmental and social situations from our discussions in chapter 15. This is not a brain region that you want to put on standby mode, but lack of sleep will force you to do that.

More Than The Sum Of The Parts

As we discussed in the introductory chapter, there is a very different set of behavioral and physiological responses to total sleep deprivation (e.g. no sleep one night) when compared to chronic sleep curtailment (e.g. sleeping 1-2 hours per night below our optimal level for several days or longer). Losing a little here and there can have some sneaky, almost sinister effects on our daytime performance.

The behavioral consequences of partial sleep loss add up over time and cause deficits in behavioral performance that are the same as total sleep deprivation for one to three nights. Restricted sleep has a variety of affects on cognitive performance, but most profoundly influences behavioral alertness. Performance on psychomotor tasks that require vigilant attention are very sensitive to sleep loss in general and sleep restriction in particular. These decrements get steadily worse when nightly sleep duration is restricted to between 3 and 7 hours per night.

Further, a person will experience similar reductions in the number of things that they can pay attention to at any given time, when experiencing several days of sleep restriction. This also shows a progressive loss of function in relation to the amount of sleep lost each night. The bummer about this whole situation is that catching up on sleep on the weekend isn't really effective.

Another difference between total sleep deprivation and chronic sleep curtailment is that the feelings of sleepiness do not parallel the decreases in performance. In total sleep deprivation, say you miss one night of sleep, your 'feelings' of sleepiness will be in line with your decrease in vigilance and cognitive performance. What is sneaky about chronic sleep curtailment is that your 'feelings' of sleepiness do not closely follow the decreases in performance that you will experience. So the red-flag of feeling sleepy won't be there, but your ability to pay attention will be decreased as will your ability to process and recall information. But wait, it gets sneakier still! Remember that sleep deprivation has its most profound effects on the learning and memory of new skills or knowledge. Those things that you've done a lot, that become reflexive in a sense, you still perform accurately, even in a sleep deprived state. So unless you're really paying attention or in the business of trying to learn and integrate new facts and ideas, then your decreased performance may go unnoticed.

So who cares? If we can still do all the things we need to do that we're already good at, why does this matter? If you were sitting alone in a chair with minimal interaction from your environment it probably wouldn't matter, but life isn't a spectator sport. You have to recognize and respond to a variety of environmental and social situations in your day-to-day life and this is where your SOS will become noticeable. Essentially, this puts a major damper on your ability to learn and grow. If you plan to stay stagnant for the rest of your life and have all the skills required for your happiness, then don't worry about it. But if you still have some livin' to do, get some rest, you'll need it.

What About The Children?

Ah, those crazy kids. One would think that they have limitless amounts of energy (teenagers excluded, of course), but the fact of the matter is that kids' sleep needs are substantial. Sleep is critical for optimal physical growth and development, and invaluable for their brain development as well. Although duration of sleep tends to decrease as kids move from grade-school into high-school, sleep-research indicates that the sleep needs of teenagers are still 9-10 hours per night, even though they may not get that. Teens tend to get much less sleep than they need. There are many potential reasons for this. The window of self-regulated sleep decreases during the teen years. Kids have a lot of stuff that they can do that will keep them up to all hours of the night. However, this is in conflict with the early start times of many schools. Everything we know about teenage physiology suggests that they really shouldn't be forced to get up so early for high school but we also need to make efforts to get them to bed earlier.

Some interesting studies show that we should also attempt to keep their 'weekend shift' to a minimum. Kids may go to bed at a reasonable hour during the school week, but then stay up all hours on the weekend. Teens who 'shift' 2 hours or less (meaning their weekend bed and rise time is within 2 hours of their school week routine) get better grades in school. Some of this likely relates to other factors, but some also relates to the physiology of their circadian rhythms. Bouncing back and forth between school week and weekend bedtimes is not good for their cognitive function.

In addition to their own health and cognitive performance, you should consider the poor parents in the equation as well. There are plenty of data out there showing the effects of sleep deprivation on the parent's of newborns to indicate that their good sleep may be your good sleep. All parents can relate to this. For older children and adolescents the issue may not be interruption of your sleep, per say, but having to deal with a sleep-deprived, hormonally crazed individual with a yet-to-be-developed frontal cortex.

For younger kids, a good strategy is to work with set bedtimes to ensure they are getting the amount of sleep that they need. For teenagers, this strategy may not work as easily. One approach that might be less authoritarian would be to challenge your teen to try out a more optimal-sleep situation for a couple weeks and see if they notice the difference. Make sure they keep some kind of record (i.e. journal, blog, video diary, something) so you can keep a record of how they felt before they started your challenge and then how they felt after they have stuck to the challenge for a couple weeks. If they are resistant to taking the challenge you could always incentivize the challenge by offering a reward for successfully completing the agreed upon duration of optimal-sleep. We realize this isn't a trivial task to attempt with teenagers, but there may be hope. Tracking systems that require less "effort" may be right around the corner. Even the Nintendo Wii has a log sheet that keeps track of what days an individual has used the entertainment system, what games they have played and for how long. Maybe the folks at Nintendo can come up with a clever sleep-promoting game? Well, maybe not.

Moving On

We've come to the end of our section on sleep and how it affects the brain. Next we will recap our discussions in the summary section to highlight the major points and send you off with some customized action plans to help you incorporate the four brain fitness cornerstones into your routine and boost your EPIC performance.

SUCCESSFUL SLEEPING SUMMARY

Hopefully we've been able to convey the importance of sleep and bring to your attention how easily we can cheat ourselves out of the sleep we deserve. Remember that this is a critical, and very active part of your life, and if you don't give sleep its due time you'll be withdrawing from your reserves faster than you can make deposits from the other cornerstones. Here we'll summarize some of the key topics from this section and provide a few action points.

Key Concepts:

- Sleep is a very productive part of your life, it is not time wasted.
- Everyone's sleep needs are unique.
- Losing a little sleep each night has very sneaky unwanted effects on your health.
- SOS causes you to respond in appropriately to stressful and emotional events.
- SOS can have dramatic effects on your body and your brain.
- SOS hinders your ability to learn and remember.
- Sleeping in on the weekend can't make up for chronic sleep loss.

Key Action Points:

- Assess your sleep behavior. Are you giving yourself the opportunity and the permission to sleep?

- Determine your sleep needs. In a perfect world, what would be your optimal, uninterrupted, sleep duration? Now, prioritize at least that amount of time for sleep.
- Determine your sleep hygiene. Are there environmental or behavioral steps that you can take?
- Is the sleep problem really yours? SOS of a partner or child may negatively affect your sleep. Remember many times their good sleep is your good sleep.
- If you are unable to address your sleep issues on your own, seek the help of a professional. There are many clinical and technological possibilities that can help you get the sleep you deserve.

Neural Nugget #6 – Ice Cream Socials

We've interjected comments about the benefits of supportive social networks in many chapters throughout this book. However, due to the importance of this topic, it deserves its own neural nugget. Social networks are hugely important for several different aspects of promoting and maintaining life-long brain fitness.

First, in order to maintain any healthy behavioral change and incorporate new habits into your life, you would greatly benefit being accountable to someone. A very small percentage of people can successfully hold themselves accountable and stick to a plan. The vast majority of us need someone else to lean on, bounce ideas off, vent to or just have them kick us in the butt every now and then, whether it's sticking to a good diet, exercising regularly, or whatever. Accountability is huge. Accountability partners provide motivation and direction for each other. If you don't have anyone who can act in this capacity for you, find someone on-line. In the resources section of this book we have listed a few good places to start or maybe you already have your favorite websites. Personal interaction is probably better but internet interactions can be beneficial as well.

Second, social support groups can help you work through problems you're having, whether psychological or physical. You're not alone in this world. No matter what bad experiences you've had, there are likely other folks out there going through the same stuff and you can find them. Sometimes support groups are formal gatherings, lead by a therapist or counselor. Other times they are less formal and just meet to exchange stories and provide support. These groups can provide a huge amount of stress relief, which especially helps your EQ, or emotional intelligence; and if you've read this book you know that can feedback to improve your physical and cognitive health as well.

Third, even if you don't have specific issues that benefit from group type therapies, or have problems sticking to a health plan, surrounding yourself with friends has enormous brain benefits. Many studies show that regular leisure activities are associated with greater cognitive fitness in your older years. We talked about some of these in chapters 10 and 13 already. Social interactions can come in almost any form, from bridge clubs to book clubs to tennis clubs; and from attending art fairs to concerts in the park to the opera. The bottom line is to stay engaged in life and do it with other people. We are social animals and our brains are built for social interaction.

You can view social support as the bedrock that all the other four cornerstones rest on. The more solid and stable the bedrock is the more stable each of the cornerstones will be and the better you will be able to build a strong framework of life-long brain fitness.

Connecting Cornerstones

EPIC Performance

CHAPTER 18

WRAP IT UP – AND TAKE IT

One Week Action Plan (then another week, and another week, and another week, etc.)

"The road to success is dotted with many tempting parking places."

- Will Rogers (comedian and actor)

You've seen them before. "The 30-day weight loss plan". "Three weeks to perfect abs and buns". "Nine weeks to a better memory". We like plans and time frames put on those plans. We're going to offer you one here, but with a caveat right up front. If you want to take advantage of all the stuff we've laid out throughout this book to improve your brain function and boost you EPIC performance, you're going to have to incorporate life-long habits. Technically "the rest of your life" is a time-frame.

Think about taking a shower. In just a few minutes, you can completely turn your attitude around, feel refreshed and smell like an Irish spring. But if you want to feel like that tomorrow, you have to take another shower. You can't just take one shower and remain clean for the rest of your life. Fitness is the same. You don't work hard for several months, get fit, and then say "OK, now I can stop working out". No. You need to keep going. Brain fitness is no different; it's a journey, not a destination. We want your journey to be fun, enjoyable, clear *and* full of vibrant health. If you view the four cornerstones of brain fitness for what they are, fundamental habits to improve your brain health, then you're on the right road.

In this chapter, we'll promise to help you develop a plan, but you have to promise not to see it as a something you adopt for a finite period of time and then go back to your old ways of doing things. Like we mentioned before, the best definition of insanity is 'doing things the same way you have always done them and expecting different results'. Will it be difficult? Well, that's up to you. If you ask people who have been living a healthy lifestyle for some time if it's difficult, they'll most certainly so no. In fact, the more you adopt healthy habits, the easier *and* more enjoyable they become.

In chapter 4, we discussed how you can adjust your brain to actually crave healthy behaviors. Once you start down this road and your brain figures out that living healthy makes you feel great, your reward centers will light up for good food, exercise, sleep and mental challenges. You will crave the things that improve your brain fitness, which will send you into an upward spiral. It's an amazing thing that you have to experience for yourself.

So let's get started. We'll integrate the major points of each of the four cornerstones and help you set up a method to find what you like and what works for you. We'll help you embark on your own ACTION plan (you didn't honestly think you'd get through the final chapter without a good acronym), which has the following six steps:

1. Assess (where you are now).
2. Commit (to achieving your goals).
3. Tackle (your first steps).
4. Incorporate (habits into your lifestyle).
5. Observe (what's working and what's not).
6. Navigate (continually towards your goals).

The First Day – Get The Laundry List

We'll start with a list of stuff that you'll need in order to take full advantage of this chapter, which we highly recommend you do. Maybe you already have these, if not, go get em'.

Pocket Journal (less than $10)
Pedometer (less than $10)
Sport Watch or Stopwatch (less than $30)
Good pair of walking/running shoes ($40 - $80)

Step 1 – Assess (where you are now)

Every good plan must start with an assessment. If you don't know where you're at or where you want to be, you can't possibly figure out the route to get there. What you need to do is pull out that compass and figure out exactly where you are. In this step, you'll do some monitoring of your current eating, exercise, mental workouts and sleep routines. You can read through this section completely and then go back and do all of these self-evaluations at the same time over the next few days.

Before you get into taking any action regarding increasing your physical activity, you should head to the doc for a complete physical. This will (hopefully) give you the go ahead and serve as a baseline measure for all the standard blood work and other health indicators.

Nutrition Tracker

Before you start tracking what you're eating, open up your cupboards and fridge and just take a visual survey. How much of the stuff in there would you lump into the 'healthy' category and how much would you call 'junk food'? Just look at it for a minute. Let the image settle into your brain. This is your starting point. Maybe you don't eat all that stuff. Maybe it's your spouse or your kids. But this exercise is for them too. Everyone has the right to a fit brain.

The first thing you want to do is to track the important components of what you're putting in your mouth. This is not meant to be an exact science but to give you an honest idea of what you're actually eating. It's up to you how long you want to track meals for and how much effort you want to put into this. However, we suggest diligence for at least 3 days. Grab that pocket diary you bought and make a list of the following categories that looks like this, with a smiley face at the top:

☺

1. Fruits
2. Vegetables
3. Good Fats
4. Fiber
5. Protein
6. Calcium
7. Multi-Vitamin / Mineral

Now make another short list with a frowning face at the top like this:

☹

1. Bad Fats
2. High Sugar
3. Excess Alcohol

If you really want to get fancy, you can use an on-line tracking system. Just do a search for 'free diet journal' and you'll find several good ones.

OK. To keep it simple, you're just going to put a little check mark next to each item when you eat a food with that in it. Keep track of each day separately. No calorie counting or fancy formulas, there are plenty of good books and resources out there if you want to get into that level of detail. We want to help you decide whether or not you're putting brain friendly foods in your mouth on a regular basis. However, in order to do a good job at tracking your nutritional intake you're going to have to learn a few basics about reading nutrition labels, so let's go though these categories so you know how to track them.

Fruits and Vegetables. Put a check next to these every time you eat a serving, which is about ½ cup raw fruits or veggies or 1 cup cooked veggies.

Good Fats. For packaged foods, you'll need to pull this information off the food labels. First, look at the fat content. The label shows you total fat, saturated fat and trans fat. If you subtract the saturated and trans fat from the total fat, you're left with 'good fats', which are poly- and mono-unsaturated fats. Some labels may even list these directly. So if you see 16 grams of fat on a label but only 2 grams of saturated fat, don't freak out! That means there are 14 grams of good fat in there. Put a check mark next for every serving of good fat, which you can consider about 15 grams, which is about what you get from a handful of nuts, a piece of fatty fish (not fried), or a cup of legumes.

Fiber. You'll find this information on carbohydrate part of the label. Put a check for every serving of fiber, which is about 5 grams. Also consider a serving of fruits or vegetables a serving of fiber as well.

Protein. This is also listed directly on the label. Put a check for each serving, which is about 15 grams. If you're eating meat that didn't come with a label, a serving is 3-4 ounces, or about the size of the palm of your hand (much less than many people think is a serving).

Calcium. Again, you can get this right on the label, except it's probably listed as a '%' instead of in grams. Put a check for every serving, which is about 30%. You'll get this amount from a cup of milk, soy milk or an ounce of cheese.

Multi-Vitamin / Mineral. Put a check if you took the full dose of your multi-vitamin and mineral complex. If you don't currently take one, check the resources section for what to look for in a product and some recommendations.

Bad Fats. These are saturated and trans fats. Put a check next to 'bad fats' for every serving, which is about 5 grams. Put a big red X with a skull and crossbones every time you eat anything with trans fats, because these should be avoided completely. But you can't just trust the label on this if it says 0g. You have to look at the ingredients for partially hydrogenated oils. If this is in the ingredients, the food has trans fats. If it contains less than 0.5g per serving the label will say 0g. It's still bad.

High sugar. Sugar is listed directly on the label under carbohydrates. This is a little bit of a tough one. The goal is to eat low glycemic foods, which you can't really tell directly from the label. For our purposes, as a rule of thumb, put a check for every serving of food (or drink) that has more than 20 grams of sugar AND less than 40 grams of total carbohydrate. If the product actually lists the glycemic index, which is happening more and more, then put a check for foods that have an index of 70 or greater.

Excess Alcohol. You can find experts on both sides of the fence when it comes to alcohol. However, most of the data suggest that 1-2 drinks per day for men and 1 drink per day for women is OK or potentially beneficial for your heart (which usually means good for your brain). So put a check next to this if you drink more than that on any given day.

OK. After a few days tracking, go back and look at your notes.

Here's what you want to see for the good stuff:

5-9 checks of fruits and vegetables (total). Hopefully they're not all in the fruits or all in the vegetables but spread across the two. Optimal these will come from eating a variety of colors and types of these foods.

4-5 checks of good fats. Optimally, this will contain some fish for the brain health omega-3s, as shown on the chart in chapter 3.

5-6 checks for fiber. Optimally these should come from whole grains, fruits, vegetables and legumes.

5-6 checks for protein. Optimally these will be from low or healthy fat sources, like chicken, fish, soy or extra low fat beef.

Here's what you want to see for the bad stuff:

0-2 checks for bad fats. It's impossible to avoid saturated fat completely. However, if you're getting more than this then you're getting too many of your calories from bad fat. If you have *any* trans fats in your diet, these really should go.

0-1 checks for high sugar. You really want to make a substantial effort to get high glycemic foods out of your diet. The occasional treat in moderation is OK, but not every day.

How did you do? Was it better or worse than you thought? Either way, it's the truth, and that will set you free.

Exercise / Physical Activity Tracker

You're going to want to track your physical activity in a couple of different ways. First, (and very easy) is to strap on that pedometer that you bought and simply track your steps for several days. At the end of each day, you can write down how many steps you put in from the time you got up, to the time you went to bed. You'll want to keep the pedometer on your night stand so that you can put it on as soon as you get up. Just transfer it from your PJs to your work clothes to whatever you wear at home (if you're in the habit of running around the house naked, you're just going to have to carry it).

Second, you'll want to track how much time you spend actually exercising or doing something that really gets your heart rate up, like digging ditches or chasing your dog around. You want to know how much activity you're getting, in addition to your steps. This is especially important if you're cycling, swimming, or doing some other activity that won't register on your pedometer as steps. You still want to get credit for that time. We wouldn't recommend wearing your pedometer in the pool anyway.

So, you'll write down your steps and your time spent with an elevated heart rate due to moderate physical activity or exercise (an increased heart rate watching *Bay Watch* doesn't count). After several 'normal' days take a look at your notes and see if you meet the following benchmarks.

Minimally, you should find that you move around in a way that gets your heart rate a little elevated for at least a 20 minute stretch, three days per week. You should also find yourself at least hitting about 5,000 steps (which is half the optimal) on most days. If you're not hitting those marks, you're likely entering PADS, which you'll remember as physical activity deficiency syndrome.

Optimally, you should be engaging in about 30 minute bouts of exercise on most days and hitting 10,000 steps per day, but remember these goals don't need to be achieved immediately. If you average 2000 steps a day, don't make 10,000 your goal for next week. A good short-term goal would be to average 2200 steps per day, and build from there. Of course, if you're working out in ways that won't register pedometer steps then you shouldn't really worry about the steps as much. Someone who averages 2000 steps per day, but is logging 500 miles a week training for the Tour de France, shouldn't fret over their step count. However, walking regularly is still a great activity, whether or not you're working out by other means.

How did you do? Are you hitting the marks, or could you use some improvement in the area of physical activity and exercise? Keep this in mind when we get to step 2, on committing yourself.

Mental Activity Tracker

Unless you are participating in a structured mental activity program, this behavior will be a bit trickier to track. However, you can do it by paying attention to your actions throughout your day. Again, you'll want to keep that pocket journal handy for notes. Write down a list of the following five categories that you'll check off as you find yourself participating in:

1. Routine tasks
2. New experiences
3. Challenging activities
4. Reflective relaxation
5. Social interaction

A good way to track your activity involvement in these different aspects of mental activity is to set your watch to beep every hour and then just make a check mark next to the one you spent the most time in during that previous hour. If you do this for a few days you'll get a feeling for how much your really engaging in this important brain fitness cornerstone. First, let's define these a little further:

Routine tasks are something you've done a bunch of times and don't really need to think about, like, laundry housework or mundane tasks on the job. It also includes passive activities, like watching TV.

New experiences are obviously something you haven't done before. It may or may not be too difficult or challenging, but it at least requires learning something at some level or taking a different perspective. For example, learning a new role at work or going to see Phantom of the Opera if you've never been to the opera before.

Challenging activities require some mental effort and thinking. This could be figuring out problems at work, coaching a sports team that requires constant strategery (we can thank Saturday Night Live's portrayal of G.W.B. for that word), reading something educational or doing challenging puzzles. Doing the daily crossword doesn't count if you do it every day and it's too easy. Doing the *New York Times* crossword that really requires some time and effort, would be OK.

Reflective relaxation includes things like meditation, midnfulness, Tai Chi or Yoga that we discussed in chapter 12.

Social interactions are also obvious. This is either leisure time with friends or work related activities that require a group effort where you must work positively with other people.

You get the idea. Every hour, just make a quick check mark next to the type of activity you spent your time doing. Activities may fall into multiple categories so just make your check marks next to whatever applies. After a few days, review your notes and see what kinds of activities are taking up most of your time.

How did you do? Are you doing something new or challenging on most days? We all will spend a big chunk of time doing mundane tasks, that's part of life, but we should get plenty of activity in the other categories as well in order to challenge or mind and build those brain connections on a regular basis.

Sleep Tracker

Tracking your sleep shouldn't be too difficult. It won't have all the bells, whistles and buzzers available in a clinical sleep lab, but you should be sure to track a few things: The hours you devoted to sleep, the hours you feel you actually slept, and a general measure of whether or not you had a good night's sleep. You probably already have a fairly good idea about how many hours you sleep and how often you sleep well, but let's go through the exercise just to make sure. Make a note in your pocket journal every morning when you got up to determine the duration and quality of your sleep. After several days take a look and see how you're doing.

Are you getting the number of hours that you feel you need? Are you having problems sleeping on a regular basis?

Understanding your starting point for all the cornerstones is critical in order to decide where you need to pay more attention in your life. Now that you have a good idea, let's figure out goals you want to work toward and what habits you'll need to replace in order to do that.

Step 2 – Commit (to achieving your goals)

In order to commit to achieving any kind of healthy behavioral change, you have to relate that change to helping you accomplish something you really want. You are not going to make any sustainable changes in your life just because your friends, spouse, doctor or some book told you it would be good for you. You have to convince yourself that these healthy changes are something that you want. Hopefully, this book has given you plenty of reasons to do that.

In this step, you'll design your goals as to where you want to be and commit yourself to getting there. Everyone has different levels of desired achievement, so there's no 'one plan fits all' here. We are assuming, since your reading this book that you want to get and stay emotionally, physically and cognitively healthy. But you first have to define what that means to you and what it would enable you to accomplish. Some goals are easy to measure while others are less tangible. Take a minute to define some specific goals and write them down.

Weight loss goals are easy to measure. If you want to weigh 135 pounds, you just get on the scale and see how close you are. You can also measure many fitness goals. Maybe you want to walk a mile without resting, or run a marathon. Some intellectual goals, like learning to play the piano proficiently, learning to speak Chinese, or mastering counting into a six-shoe card deck to beat the odds in Vegas also have measurable values. However, many aspects of brain health just aren't that easy to measure. Yes, you can take memory tests and other types of cognitive performance tests and watch yourself improve. But as we discussed in chapter 13, many of these skills aren't easy to generalize to everyday life. One brain health goal that we all seek is to live a cognitively vibrant life until the end and stave off any form of dementia. Some of your goals will be measurable while other will be less tangible, but write them out as clearly as you can.

Throughout this book, we have given you many approaches using the four cornerstones of brain fitness to boost your odds of life-long brain health. You can also use many of these approaches to pursue measurable physical and cognitive health goals. Look back at your self-assessment in the previous step and associate what your current habits are doing to your odds of achieving life-long brain health or your more tangible goals. Ask yourself which healthy habits you need to add and which poor habits you need to replace, in order to reach your goals.

It's important to look at good and bad habits in pairs because it's much easier to replace a bad habit with a good one, than to just drop a bad habit alone. Identify specific areas of your diet, your physical activity, your mental activity and your sleep habits that you want to change. Some examples of habit pairs are to eat more vegetables and less dessert; increase your daily number of steps and watch less TV; increase your exposure to new experiences and reduce redundancy in your life; or go to bed earlier and stop watching late night TV so often. All of these will increase your odds of boosting brain fitness. To achieve a specific goal, like running a marathon for example, you would need to adopt specific diet, exercise and sleep habits as well. What do you need to do differently to get what you want?

A central tenet of human psychology is that we always behave in a way to seek pleasure or avoid pain. A good way to commit to your specific brain health goals is to associate each new habit that you want to adopt with seeking pleasure; and each old habit you want to replace with avoiding pain. To do this, take out your pocket journal and write at the top of the page a habit you want to adopt, then describe in vivid detail what this new habit would do for you. How would it make you feel? How would it add vibrancy to your life and the lives of those around you? See, smell and taste the results of your new healthy habit. Akin to this, write down a habit you want to replace on the top of another page and write out the consequences of not replacing this habit. How would it slowly degrade your health or increase your odds for poor brain fitness as you age? What would that do to the people around you? Repeat this for each of the habits you want to adopt and replace. This very powerful technique will help you commit to the changes that you want to make.

Step 3 – Tackle (your first steps)

Sometimes getting started is the hardest part. You may be moving into unknown territory. Or perhaps, you're embarking on a road that you've tried to go down before and couldn't stick to. After finishing step two, you may even look at some of your goals and re-evaluate whether or not you can really achieve them. A great way to tackle big goals in any area is to chunk them down using a technique called mind-mapping.

With mind-mapping you'll write your goal in a circle in the middle of a piece of paper. Then, in smaller circles surrounding your goal (like spokes coming out of a wheel hub), write all the major steps you need to do in order to achieve it. Now, take those steps and break them down even further until you have something very small and simple that you can do right away. You want to scale your milestones so that you have smaller stepping-stones of success that will help you climb towards your larger goals. Unless you are Superman, it's pretty hard to leap a tall building in a single bound, but almost anyone can get to the top if you take the stairs.

For example, let's say you have the goal to run a marathon. That's a big goal for many people. You would take the goal 'run a marathon' and write it in a circle in the middle of a piece of paper. What does it take to wake up one day ready to run a marathon? You would identify several things you would need to accomplish to in order to prepare for a marathon and write those in smaller circles around the big goal. You would have to follow a training plan, eat energy rich and nutritious foods, sleep well to allow for recovery, and probably find someone to provide moral support for your efforts for several months, maybe even a few years. Let's take just one of those steps, follow a training plan, and break it down further. What can you do right now? How about buy some running shoes, buy a book with a tried and true marathon training plan, and make an appointment with your doctor to get a physical and clearance to begin? Those are all things you can do today and you're now on your way to achieving that goal. Then you just need to follow the steps laid out before you until you reach your destination. Reaching every big goal is just a series of smaller steps, that, when broken down are not too daunting. Are you guaranteed success if you follow the plan? Of course not. But you are guaranteed no success if you don't try.

As we said in the very beginning of this book, many of us today will live into our 80s, 90s or even 100s. How much life do you have left? Why not live it pursuing what you really want to achieve. Thomas Edison said, *"If we do all the things we are capable of doing we would literally astound ourselves"*

With the first step behind you, let's move on.

Step 4 – Integrate (habits into your lifestyle)

Any goal worth achieving will require some effort into incorporating new habits into your life. That's really what our goal is with this book. To help you identify and incorporate habits into your life that will keep you *BrainFit*. In step 1, you identified where you're starting from. In step 2, you identified where you're going, and the types of habits you need in order to get there. In step 3, you started to take action. In this step, you'll solidify the incorporation of those habits into your life.

Getting started on a goal and continuing to make progress is a great motivator. However, there will be periods where you don't seem to make any progress, even with continued effort. During these times, you really need to stay focused on where you are going in order to maintain the psychological momentum. A great way to do this is to review your goals on a daily basis. You can just pull out your journal, read your top goals on each page, the reasons you want to achieve them and the habits you must adopt to get you there. This helps you stay on track and integrates an easy daily activity into your routine. Reviewing your goals works best first thing in the morning and last thing in the evening. The morning review gets your day started with focus and the evening review puts your goals into your head just before going to sleep.

You can incorporate the healthy habits needed for your success into your life, just like brushing your teeth. No matter which of the cornerstones you are currently focusing on adopting a healthy habit for, you can eventually make it automatic. In Jack Canfield's book, *The Success Principles*, he has one section titled "99% is a Bitch, 100% is a Breeze". What he highlights with this discussion is that true habits that you do all the time are easy. It's when you allow yourself to forgo the behavior under 'special circumstance' that makes it tough. You don't spend every night debating with yourself whether or not you really need to brush your teeth at night, you just do it. OK, sometimes you may forget, but it's truly a habit.

You can make eating a good breakfast or walking 30 minutes first thing in the morning an equally strong habit. You just have to commit 100% and put yourself on automatic. However, you also want to give yourself a fighting chance. Committing to getting out of bed and walking down into the basement to get on the treadmill for 30 minutes is very different than committing yourself to walking outside if you live in a part of the world that experiences sub-freezing temperatures half the year. Not that you couldn't do it in harsher conditions, but be reasonable. Work within your own tendencies to give yourself the best possible chance at success.

In addition to incorporating life style habits that you identified in step 2, you'll want to continue to make progress towards your goals by acting on the small steps you mapped out in step 3. You should have broken your bigger goals into small easier steps that you can act on every day. Review your mind map each morning, pick your next step or steps and make it happen. Reviewing your daily progress is a great way to keep yourself moving. You may not realize how far you've come until one day you look back to see what you have already accomplished.

You could walk from New York to Los Angeles, even if you could only walk one mile per day. It would take you seven and a half years to do it, but you would eventually get there. Integrate your most important health habits and you'll reach amazing goals.

Step 5 – Observe (what's working and what's not)

Things change. Life is a very dynamic process. Sometimes adjustments are needed in order to achieve your biggest goals. Maybe you tried a diet plan that just doesn't seem to be working for you. You shouldn't continue on blindly just because you started down that road. If your goal is to lose weight and keep it off you need to find the best plan for your metabolism, tastes and preferences. This may require some reevaluation and adjustment as you go. Maybe that 6:30 am walk just isn't working for you and you tend to feel much better and stick to it easier when you walk right after work at 6:00 pm. You will get to know your own strengths and weaknesses as you progress toward your goal. Always play to your strengths for the best chance at success.

With that said, you also need to stick with a plan long enough to give it a chance. If you're trying a new diet, give it at least several weeks, if not months to really test it out. There will be an adjustment period in adopting any lifestyle changes and health habits. If you started lifting weights, you wouldn't quit on the first day just because you couldn't bench the whole stack. Things take time.

Related to this point, don't quit on something just because you messed up once. If you find yourself gorging down half a cheese cake the week after you started a new diet plan, that doesn't mean you should abandon the whole plan. There is a big difference between messing up and giving up. We all mess up. You can't go through life without messing up. You will have moments of weakness where you completely abandon your diet and exercise plans, but don't quit. Get up and get back on them. Continually review the reasons why you want what you want and start again. If your reasons are strong enough then nothing will stop you.

Step 6 – Navigate (continually toward your goals)

Nobody goes from point A to point B in a straight line, even though that's the shortest distance. There are always adjustments to make during the course. When a plane takes off from New York's JFK airport for LAX in Los Angeles, the pilots, crew and all the passengers know exactly where they're going. But during the flight the plane will make hundreds of small adjustments due to wind speed, turbulence, storms to avoid, etc. There are always challenges on the way on any trip that require navigational adjustment.

The same will be true when moving toward your goals. This type of navigation is different than observing what's working and what's not as you did in step 5. This type of navigation keeps your eye on your goal, realizing that you will face many challenges in pursuing it. Yes, you need to evaluate what's working and what's not. You also need to realize there will be setbacks, even if you are following the perfect plan. If life were too easy, it would be boring. Enjoy the journey.

About Simon & Paul

Dr. Simon Evans and Dr. Paul Burghardt are research scientists at the University of Michigan. Simon is in the Department of Psychiatry and Paul is in the Molecular and Behavioral Neuroscience institute. Both are affiliated with the UM's Comprehensive Depression Center and the Michigan Metabolomics and Obesity Center.

Simon holds a PhD in molecular biology with 15 years research and teaching experience in neuroscience. He also holds membership in the Society for Neuroscience, the American Society for Nutrition, and the American Heart Association. He is the author of dozens of scientific publications on stress, depression and brain function. Coach Simon also has a 25-year history working with youth sports and holds a national coaching license from the United States Soccer Federation. Simon lives with his wife and children in southeastern Michigan

Paul earned a MS in exercise physiology and a PhD in biomedical science and has a decade of research experience investigating how physical activity alters behavior and neurobiology. He is a member of the Society for Neuroscience and the International Behavioral Neuroscience Society. He has authored several scientific publications on response to exercise, has clinical experience investigating the effects of nutritional supplements on performance in athletes, and experience in cardiac rehabilitation programs. Coach Paul has also instructed athletes in national junior judo competitions and worked as a personal trainer. Paul also lives with his wife and child in southeastern Michigan.

Interested in having Drs. Evans and Burghardt speak to your group? Contact them at www.brainfitforlife.com.

RESOURCES

For updated resources and live links to more information, check:
http://www.brainfitforlife.com/resources

WEBSITES

General Health Websites

www.brainfitforlife.com (resources supporting this book)
www.glycemicindex.com (glycemic index help and advice)
www.fitday.com (on-line diet and exercise tracker)
www.my-calorie-counter.com (on-line diet tracker)
www.sparkpeople.com (healthy living resources)
www.acsm.org (American College of Sports Medicine)
www.exerciseismedicine.org (exercise resources)
www.diabetes.org (American Diabetes Association)
lpi.orst.edu (Linus Pauling Institute for Micronutrient Research)
www.thenutritioncode.com (Usana Health Sciences nutritionals)

Social Networking Websites

www.eons.com (social network for people 50 and over)
www.boomj.com (social network for baby boomers)
www.disaboom.com (social network for people with a disability)

Brain Fitness Websites

www.sharpbrains.com (brain fitness industry information)
www.sfn.org (Society for Neuroscience)
www.nimh.nih.gov (National Institute of Mental Health)
www.aarp.org/health/brain (AARP brain health area)
www.cdc.gov/aging/healthybrain.htm (Healthy Brain Initiative)
www.alz.org (Alzheimer's Association)
www.parkinson.org (National Parkinson Foundation)

www.nationalsleepfoundation.org (National Sleep Foundation)
www.depressioncenter.org (mood disorder resources)

RECOMMENDED FURTHER READING

Books

<u>General Health</u>

Brand Miller, J., K. Foster-Powell, and J. McMillan-Price, *The low GI diet cookbook : 100 simple, delicious smart-carb recipes, the proven way to lose weight and eat for lifelong health.* 2005, New York, N.Y.: Marlowe. 175 p.

Breus, M., *Good night : the sleep doctor's 4-week program to better sleep and better health.* 2006, New York, N.Y.: Penguin Group. viii, 324 p.

Douglas, B., *The complete idiot's guide to T'ai Chi and QiGong : illustrated.* 3rd ed. 2005, Indianapolis: Alpha Books. xxiv, 322 p.

Evans, SJ. *Brain fitness: A recipe for feeding your child's dreams and unlocking their maximum brain power.* 2006, New York, NY: Morgan James Publishing. 176 p.

Grant-Gray, J., *The sleep book : a bedside companion.* 2000, Santa Monica, CA: Aero U.S. 224 p.

Holford, P., *The new optimum nutrition bible.* Rev & updated. ed. 2005, Berkeley, Calif.: Crossing Press. xii, 576 p.

Kabat-Zinn, J. and University of Massachusetts Medical Center/Worcester. Stress Reduction Clinic., *Full catastrophe living : using the wisdom of your body and mind to face stress, pain, and illness.* Delta trade pbk. reissue. ed. 2005, New York, N.Y.: Delta Trade Paperbacks. xxxiii, 471 p.

MacWilliam, L., *Nutrisearch comparative guide to nutritional supplements: A compendium of over 1500 products available in the United States and Canada.* Nutrisearch Corporation ed. 2007, Vernon: Northern Dimensions Publishing. viii, 187p.

Oz, M., *You staying young : the owner's manual for extending your warranty.* 1st Free Press hardcover ed. 2007, New York: Free Press. xiii, 415 p.

Roizen, M.F., M. Oz, and G. Hallgren, *You-- the owner's manual : an insider's guide to the body that will make you healthier and younger.* 1st ed. 2005, New York: HarperResource. xiii, 417 p.

Sapolsky, R.M., *Why zebras don't get ulcers / Robert M. Sapolsky.* 3rd ed. 2004, New York: Times Books. xv, 539 p.

Weil, A., *Healthy aging : a lifelong guide to your physical and spiritual well-being.* 1st Knopf ed. 2005, New York: Alfred A. Knopf. 293 p.

Woodruff, S.L., *The good carb cookbook : secrets of eating low on the glycemic index.* 2001, New York: Avery. 312 p.

Brain Fitness

Doidge, N., *The brain that changes itself : stories of personal triumph from the frontiers of brain science.* 2007, New York: Viking. xvi, 427 p.

Gediman, C., *Brainfit : 10 minutes a day for a sharper mind and memory.* 2005, Nashville, Tenn.: Rutledge Hill Press. x, 307 p.

Hawkins, J. and S. Blakeslee, *On intelligence.* 1st ed. 2004, New York: Times Books. 261 p.

Holford, P., *Optimum nutrition for the mind.* 2004, Bergen, NJ: Basic Health Publications. xv, 381 p.

Kandel, E.R., *In search of memory : the emergence of a new science of mind.* 1st ed. 2006, New York: W. W. Norton & Company. xv, 510 p.

Logan, A.C., *The brain diet : the connection between nutrition, mental health, and intelligence.* Revised and expanded [ed.]. ed. 2007, Nashville, Tenn.: Cumberland House. xi, 307 p.

Lambert, K., *Lifting depression : a neuroscientist's hands-on approach to activating your brain's healing power.* 2008, New York: Basic Books. 289 p.

LeDoux, J.E., *The emotional brain : the mysterious underpinnings of emotional life.* 1996, New York: Simon & Schuster. 384 p.

LeDoux, J.E., *Synaptic self : how our brains become who we are.* 2002, New York: Viking. x, 406 p.

McEwen, B.S., *The end of stress as we know it.* 2004, Washington, D.C.: Joseph Henry Press.

Ratey, J.J. and E. Hagerman, *Spark : the revolutionary new science of exercise and the brain.* 1st ed. 2008, New York: Little, Brown. ix, 294 p.

Goal Setting and Personal Development

Canfield, J. and J. Switzer, *The success principles : how to get from where you are to where you want to be.* 1st ed. 2005, New York: Harper Resource Book. xxxiii, 473 p.
Covey, S.R., *The seven habits of highly effective people : restoring the character ethic.* 1st Fireside ed. 1990, New York: Fireside Book. 358 p.
Covey, S.R., *The 8th habit : from effectiveness to greatness.* 2006, Philadelphia, PA: Running Press.
Frankl, V.E., *Man's search for meaning.* 2006, Boston: Beacon Press. xvi, 165 p.
Gould, S.J., *The mismeasure of man.* Rev. and expanded. ed. 1996, New York: Norton. 444 p.
Tracy, B., *The psychology of achievement.* 1984, Nightingale-Conant Corp.,: Chicago, Ill.
Tracy, B., *Focal point : a proven system to simplify your life, double your productivity, and achieve all your goals.* 2002, New York: AMACOM. xii, 222 p.
Tracy, B., *Goals! : how to get everything you want-- faster than you ever thought possible.* 1st ed. 2003, San Francisco: Berrett-Koehler. xi, 289 p.
Tracy, B., *Eat that frog! : 21 great ways to stop procrastinating and get more done in less time.* 2nd ed. 2007, San Francisco, CA: Berrett-Koehler Publishers. xiv, 128 p.
Waitley, D., *Seeds of greatness : the ten best-kept secrets of total success.* 1983, Old Tappan, N.J.: Revell. 221 p.
Waitley, D., *The psychology of winning.* 1987, Nightingale-Conant Corp.,: Chicago, Ill.

The Science (in order discussed)

References for section 1 – Quality Nutrition.

Hu, Y., et al., *Relations of glycemic index and glycemic load with plasma oxidative stress markers.* Am J Clin Nutr, 2006. **84**(1): p. 70-6; quiz 266-7.
Pearce, K.L., et al., *Effect of carbohydrate distribution on postprandial glucose peaks with the use of continuous glucose*

monitoring in type 2 diabetes. Am J Clin Nutr, 2008. **87**(3): p. 638-44.

Benton, D. and S. Nabb, *Carbohydrate, memory, and mood.* Nutr Rev, 2003. **61**(5 Pt 2): p. S61-7.

Hibbeln, J.R., *Fish consumption and major depression.* Lancet, 1998. **351**(9110): p. 1213.

De Vriese, S.R., A.B. Christophe, and M. Maes, *In humans, the seasonal variation in poly-unsaturated fatty acids is related to the seasonal variation in violent suicide and serotonergic markers of violent suicide.* Prostaglandins Leukot Essent Fatty Acids, 2004. **71**(1): p. 13-8.

Huan, M., et al., *Suicide attempt and n-3 fatty acid levels in red blood cells: a case control study in China.* Biol Psychiatry, 2004. **56**(7): p. 490-6.

Sublette, M.E., et al., *Omega-3 polyunsaturated essential fatty acid status as a predictor of future suicide risk.* Am J Psychiatry, 2006. **163**(6): p. 1100-2.

Connor, S.L. and W.E. Connor, *Are fish oils beneficial in the prevention and treatment of coronary artery disease?* Am J Clin Nutr, 1997. **66**(4 Suppl): p. 1020S-1031S.

Folstein, M., et al., *The homocysteine hypothesis of depression.* Am J Psychiatry, 2007. **164**(6): p. 861-7.

Mischoulon, D. and M.F. Raab, *The role of folate in depression and dementia.* J Clin Psychiatry, 2007. **68 Suppl 10**: p. 28-33.

Williams, A.L., et al., *The role for vitamin B-6 as treatment for depression: a systematic review.* Fam Pract, 2005. **22**(5): p. 532-7.

Kaplan, B.J., et al., *Vitamins, minerals, and mood.* Psychol Bull, 2007. **133**(5): p. 747-60.

Gariballa, S. and S. Forster, *Effects of dietary supplements on depressive symptoms in older patients: a randomised double-blind placebo-controlled trial.* Clin Nutr, 2007. **26**(5): p. 545-51.

de Araujo, I.E., et al., *Food reward in the absence of taste receptor signaling.* Neuron, 2008. **57**(6): p. 930-41.

Parton, L.E., et al., *Glucose sensing by POMC neurons regulates glucose homeostasis and is impaired in obesity.* Nature, 2007. **449**(7159): p. 228-32.

Jakulj, F., et al., *A high-fat meal increases cardiovascular reactivity to psychological stress in healthy young adults.* J Nutr, 2007. **137**(4): p. 935-9.

McIntyre, R.S., et al., *Should Depressive Syndromes Be Reclassified as "Metabolic Syndrome Type II"?* Ann Clin Psychiatry, 2007. **19**(4): p. 257-64.

Luchsinger, J.A. and R. Mayeux, *Adiposity and Alzheimer's disease.* Curr Alzheimer Res, 2007. **4**(2): p. 127-34.

Wenner, M., *Infected with Insanity: Could Microbes Cause Mental Illness?* Scientific American Mind, 2008.

Boulanger, L.M. and C.J. Shatz, *Immune signalling in neural development, synaptic plasticity and disease.* Nat Rev Neurosci, 2004. **5**(7): p. 521-31.

Benton, D., A. Maconie, and C. Williams, *The influence of the glycaemic load of breakfast on the behaviour of children in school.* Physiol Behav, 2007. **92**(4): p. 717-24.

Kaplan, R.J., et al., *Cognitive performance is associated with glucose regulation in healthy elderly persons and can be enhanced with glucose and dietary carbohydrates.* Am J Clin Nutr, 2000. **72**(3): p. 825-36.

Hibbeln, J.R., et al., *Maternal seafood consumption in pregnancy and neurodevelopmental outcomes in childhood (ALSPAC study): an observational cohort study.* Lancet, 2007. **369**(9561): p. 578-85.

Judge, M.P., O. Harel, and C.J. Lammi-Keefe, *Maternal consumption of a docosahexaenoic acid-containing functional food during pregnancy: benefit for infant performance on problem-solving but not on recognition memory tasks at age 9 mo.* Am J Clin Nutr, 2007. **85**(6): p. 1572-7.

Helland, I.B., et al., *Maternal supplementation with very-long-chain n-3 fatty acids during pregnancy and lactation augments children's IQ at 4 years of age.* Pediatrics, 2003. **111**(1): p. e39-44.

Birchwood, M. and P. Trower, *The future of cognitive-behavioural therapy for psychosis: not a quasi-neuroleptic.* Br J Psychiatry, 2006. **188**: p. 107-8.

Nurk, E., et al., *Cognitive performance among the elderly and dietary fish intake: the Hordaland Health Study.* Am J Clin Nutr, 2007. **86**(5): p. 1470-8.

Sorgi, P.J., et al., *Effects of an open-label pilot study with high-dose EPA/DHA concentrates on plasma phospholipids and behavior in children with attention deficit hyperactivity disorder.* Nutr J, 2007. **6**: p. 16.

Antalis, C.J., et al., *Omega-3 fatty acid status in attention-deficit/hyperactivity disorder.* Prostaglandins Leukot Essent Fatty Acids, 2006. **75**(4-5): p. 299-308.

Young, G.S., N.J. Maharaj, and J.A. Conquer, *Blood phospholipid fatty acid analysis of adults with and without attention deficit/hyperactivity disorder.* Lipids, 2004. **39**(2): p. 117-23.

Ames, B.N., *Mitochondrial decay, a major cause of aging, can be delayed.* J Alzheimers Dis, 2004. **6**(2): p. 117-21.

Chandra, V., et al., *Incidence of Alzheimer's disease in a rural community in India: the Indo-US study.* Neurology, 2001. **57**(6): p. 985-9.

Ng, T.P., et al., *Curry consumption and cognitive function in the elderly.* Am J Epidemiol, 2006. **164**(9): p. 898-906.

Wu, A., Z. Ying, and F. Gomez-Pinilla, *Dietary curcumin counteracts the outcome of traumatic brain injury on oxidative stress, synaptic plasticity, and cognition.* Exp Neurol, 2006. **197**(2): p. 309-17.

Milgram, N.W., et al., *Acetyl-L-carnitine and alpha-lipoic acid supplementation of aged beagle dogs improves learning in two landmark discrimination tests.* Faseb J, 2007. **21**(13): p. 3756-62.

Malaguarnera, M., et al., *L-Carnitine treatment reduces severity of physical and mental fatigue and increases cognitive functions in centenarians: a randomized and controlled clinical trial.* Am J Clin Nutr, 2007. **86**(6): p. 1738-44.

D'Anci, K.E. and I.H. Rosenberg, *Folate and brain function in the elderly.* Curr Opin Clin Nutr Metab Care, 2004. **7**(6): p. 659-64.

Grodstein, F., et al., *A randomized trial of beta carotene supplementation and cognitive function in men: the Physicians' Health Study II.* Arch Intern Med, 2007. **167**(20): p. 2184-90.

Martin, A., et al., *Roles of vitamins E and C on neurodegenerative diseases and cognitive performance.* Nutr Rev, 2002. **60**(10 Pt 1): p. 308-26.

Galli, R.L., et al., *Fruit polyphenolics and brain aging: nutritional interventions targeting age-related neuronal and behavioral deficits.* Ann N Y Acad Sci, 2002. **959**: p. 128-32.

Youdim, K.A., et al., *Dietary flavonoids as potential neuroprotectants.* Biol Chem, 2002. **383**(3-4): p. 503-19.

Gonzalez-Munoz, M.J., et al., *Beer consumption reduces cerebral oxidation caused by aluminum toxicity by normalizing gene expression of tumor necrotic factor alpha and several antioxidant enzymes.* Food Chem Toxicol, 2008. **46**(3): p. 1111-8.

Letenneur, L., *Risk of dementia and alcohol and wine consumption: a review of recent results.* Biol Res, 2004. **37**(2): p. 189-93.

References for section 2 – Exercise and Physical activity.

Hoffman, M.D. and D.R. Hoffman, *Exercisers achieve greater acute exercise-induced mood enhancement than nonexercisers.* Arch Phys Med Rehabil, 2008. **89**(2): p. 358-63.

Pilu, A., et al., *Efficacy of physical activity in the adjunctive treatment of major depressive disorders: preliminary results.* Clin Pract Epidemol Ment Health, 2007. **3**: p. 8.

Strawbridge, W.J., et al., *Physical activity reduces the risk of subsequent depression for older adults.* Am J Epidemiol, 2002. **156**(4): p. 328-34.

Teri, L., et al., *Exercise plus behavioral management in patients with Alzheimer disease: a randomized controlled trial.* Jama, 2003. **290**(15): p. 2015-22.

Blumenthal, J.A., et al., *Exercise and pharmacotherapy in the treatment of major depressive disorder.* Psychosom Med, 2007. **69**(7): p. 587-96.

Martinsen, E.W., A. Hoffart, and O. Solberg, *Comparing aerobic with nonaerobic forms of exercise in the treatment of clinical depression: a randomized trial.* Compr Psychiatry, 1989. **30**(4): p. 324-31.

Dunn, A.L., et al., *Exercise treatment for depression: efficacy and dose response.* Am J Prev Med, 2005. **28**(1): p. 1-8.

Broman-Fulks, J.J., et al., *Effects of aerobic exercise on anxiety sensitivity.* Behav Res Ther, 2004. **42**(2): p. 125-36.

Broman-Fulks, J.J. and K.M. Storey, *Evaluation of a brief aerobic exercise intervention for high anxiety sensitivity.* Anxiety Stress Coping, 2008. **21**(2): p. 117-28.

Innes, K.E. and H.K. Vincent, *The influence of yoga-based programs on risk profiles in adults with type 2 diabetes mellitus: a systematic review.* Evid Based Complement Alternat Med, 2007. **4**(4): p. 469-86.

51. Sothmann, M.S., et al., *Exercise training and the cross-stressor adaptation hypothesis.* Exerc Sport Sci Rev, 1996. **24**: p. 267-87.

Wittert, G.A., et al., *Adaptation of the hypothalamopituitary adrenal axis to chronic exercise stress in humans.* Med Sci Sports Exerc, 1996. **28**(8): p. 1015-9.

Wittels, P., et al., *Aerobic fitness and sympatho-adrenal response to short-term psycho-emotional stress under field conditions.* Eur J Appl Physiol Occup Physiol, 1994. **68**(5): p. 418-24.

Cotman, C.W., N.C. Berchtold, and L.A. Christie, *Exercise builds brain health: key roles of growth factor cascades and inflammation.* Trends Neurosci, 2007. **30**(9): p. 464-72.

Balducci, S., et al., *Exercise training can modify the natural history of diabetic peripheral neuropathy.* J Diabetes Complications, 2006. **20**(4): p. 216-23.

Lemaster, J.W., et al., *Daily weight-bearing activity does not increase the risk of diabetic foot ulcers.* Med Sci Sports Exerc, 2003. **35**(7): p. 1093-9.

Smorawinski, J., et al., *Effects of three-day bed rest on metabolic, hormonal and circulatory responses to an oral glucose load in endurance or strength trained athletes and untrained subjects.* J Physiol Pharmacol, 2000. **51**(2): p. 279-89.

Goodwin, V.A., et al., *The effectiveness of exercise interventions for people with Parkinson's disease: a systematic review and meta-analysis.* Mov Disord, 2008. **23**(5): p. 631-40.

Hirsch, M.A., et al., *The effects of balance training and high-intensity resistance training on persons with idiopathic Parkinson's disease.* Arch Phys Med Rehabil, 2003. **84**(8): p. 1109-17.

Logroscino, G., et al., *Physical activity and risk of Parkinson's disease: a prospective cohort study.* J Neurol Neurosurg Psychiatry, 2006. **77**(12): p. 1318-22.

Falvo, M.J., B.K. Schilling, and G.M. Earhart, *Parkinson's disease and resistive exercise: rationale, review, and recommendations.* Mov Disord, 2008. **23**(1): p. 1-11.

Gomez-Pinilla, F., L. Dao, and V. So, *Physical exercise induces FGF-2 and its mRNA in the hippocampus.* Brain Res, 1997. **764**(1-2): p. 1-8.

van Praag, H., G. Kempermann, and F.H. Gage, *Running increases cell proliferation and neurogenesis in the adult mouse dentate gyrus.* Nat Neurosci, 1999. **2**(3): p. 266-70.

van Praag, H., et al., *Exercise enhances learning and hippocampal neurogenesis in aged mice.* J Neurosci, 2005. **25**(38): p. 8680-5.

Hillman, C.H., K.I. Erickson, and A.F. Kramer, *Be smart, exercise your heart: exercise effects on brain and cognition.* Nat Rev Neurosci, 2008. **9**(1): p. 58-65.

Winter, B., et al., *High impact running improves learning.* Neurobiol Learn Mem, 2007. **87**(4): p. 597-609.

Covassin, T., et al., *Effects of a maximal exercise test on neurocognitive function.* Br J Sports Med, 2007. **41**(6): p. 370-4; discussion 374.

Colcombe, S.J., et al., *Aerobic fitness reduces brain tissue loss in aging humans.* J Gerontol A Biol Sci Med Sci, 2003. **58**(2): p. 176-80.

Kramer, A.F., et al., *Enhancing brain and cognitive function of older adults through fitness training.* J Mol Neurosci, 2003. **20**(3): p. 213-21.

References for section 3 – Mental activity.

Zhao, C., W. Deng, and F.H. Gage, *Mechanisms and functional implications of adult neurogenesis.* Cell, 2008. **132**(4): p. 645-60.

Cameron, H.A. and A.G. Dayer, *New interneurons in the adult neocortex: small, sparse, but significant?* Biol Psychiatry, 2008. **63**(7): p. 650-5.

Kokoeva, M.V., H. Yin, and J.S. Flier, *Evidence for constitutive neural cell proliferation in the adult murine hypothalamus.* J Comp Neurol, 2007. **505**(2): p. 209-20.

Saetre, P., et al., *Inflammation-related genes up-regulated in schizophrenia brains.* BMC Psychiatry, 2007. **7**: p. 46.

Fratiglioni, L., S. Paillard-Borg, and B. Winblad, *An active and socially integrated lifestyle in late life might protect against dementia.* Lancet Neurol, 2004. **3**(6): p. 343-53.

Golkaramnay, V., et al., *The exploration of the effectiveness of group therapy through an Internet chat as aftercare: a controlled naturalistic study.* Psychother Psychosom, 2007. **76**(4): p. 219-25.

Praissman, S., *Mindfulness-based stress reduction: A literature review and clinician's guide.* J Am Acad Nurse Pract, 2008. **20**(4): p. 212-6.

Block-Lerner, J., et al., *The case for mindfulness-based approaches in the cultivation of empathy: does nonjudgmental, present-*

moment awareness increase capacity for perspective-taking and empathic concern? J Marital Fam Ther, 2007. **33**(4): p. 501-16.

Barnes, S., et al., *The role of mindfulness in romantic relationship satisfaction and responses to relationship stress.* J Marital Fam Ther, 2007. **33**(4): p. 482-500.

Williams, J.M., et al., *Mindfulness-based Cognitive Therapy (MBCT) in bipolar disorder: preliminary evaluation of immediate effects on between-episode functioning.* J Affect Disord, 2008. **107**(1-3): p. 275-9.

Evans, S., et al., *Mindfulness-based cognitive therapy for generalized anxiety disorder.* J Anxiety Disord, 2008. **22**(4): p. 716-21.

Kingston, T., et al., *Mindfulness-based cognitive therapy for residual depressive symptoms.* Psychol Psychother, 2007. **80**(Pt 2): p. 193-203.

Williams, J.M., et al., *Mindfulness-based cognitive therapy for prevention of recurrence of suicidal behavior.* J Clin Psychol, 2006. **62**(2): p. 201-10.

Singh, N.N., et al., *Mindfulness training assists individuals with moderate mental retardation to maintain their community placements.* Behav Modif, 2007. **31**(6): p. 800-14.

Zylowska, L., et al., *Mindfulness Meditation Training in Adults and Adolescents With ADHD: A Feasibility Study.* J Atten Disord, 2008. **11**(6): p. 737-46.

Kenny, M.A. and J.M. Williams, *Treatment-resistant depressed patients show a good response to Mindfulness-based Cognitive Therapy.* Behav Res Ther, 2007. **45**(3): p. 617-25.

Morone, N.E., C.M. Greco, and D.K. Weiner, *Mindfulness meditation for the treatment of chronic low back pain in older adults: a randomized controlled pilot study.* Pain, 2008. **134**(3): p. 310-9.

Grossman, P., et al., *Mindfulness training as an intervention for fibromyalgia: evidence of postintervention and 3-year follow-up benefits in well-being.* Psychother Psychosom, 2007. **76**(4): p. 226-33.

Akil, H., *Stressed and depressed.* Nat Med, 2005. **11**(2): p. 116-8.

Bedard, M., et al., *Pilot evaluation of a mindfulness-based intervention to improve quality of life among individuals who sustained traumatic brain injuries.* Disabil Rehabil, 2003. **25**(13): p. 722-31.

Price, D.D., D.G. Finniss, and F. Benedetti, *A comprehensive review of the placebo effect: recent advances and current thought.* Annu Rev Psychol, 2008. **59**: p. 565-90.

Cohen, S., et al., *Positive emotional style predicts resistance to illness after experimental exposure to rhinovirus or influenza a virus.* Psychosom Med, 2006. **68**(6): p. 809-15.

Crum, A.J. and E.J. Langer, *Mind-set matters: exercise and the placebo effect.* Psychol Sci, 2007. **18**(2): p. 165-71.

Arias, A.J., et al., *Systematic review of the efficacy of meditation techniques as treatments for medical illness.* J Altern Complement Med, 2006. **12**(8): p. 817-32.

Gordon, L.A., et al., *Effect of exercise therapy on lipid profile and oxidative stress indicators in patients with type 2 diabetes.* BMC Complement Altern Med, 2008. **8**: p. 21.

Taylor-Piliae, R.E. and W.L. Haskell, *Tai Chi exercise and stroke rehabilitation.* Top Stroke Rehabil, 2007. **14**(4): p. 9-22.

McCain, N.L., et al., *A randomized clinical trial of alternative stress management interventions in persons with HIV infection.* J Consult Clin Psychol, 2008. **76**(3): p. 431-41.

Yang, Y., et al., *Effects of a Taiji and Qigong intervention on the antibody response to influenza vaccine in older adults.* Am J Chin Med, 2007. **35**(4): p. 597-607.

Irwin, M.R., R. Olmstead, and M.N. Oxman, *Augmenting immune responses to varicella zoster virus in older adults: a randomized, controlled trial of Tai Chi.* J Am Geriatr Soc, 2007. **55**(4): p. 511-7.

Matchim, Y. and J.M. Armer, *Measuring the psychological impact of mindfulness meditation on health among patients with cancer: a literature review.* Oncol Nurs Forum, 2007. **34**(5): p. 1059-66.

Ybarra, O., et al., *Mental exercising through simple socializing: social interaction promotes general cognitive functioning.* Pers Soc Psychol Bull, 2008. **34**(2): p. 248-59.

Stern, Y., *What is cognitive reserve? Theory and research application of the reserve concept.* J Int Neuropsychol Soc, 2002. **8**(3): p. 448-60.

Lemonick, M.D. and A. Park, *The nun study. How one scientist and 678 sisters are helping unlock the secrets of Alzheimer's.* Time, 2001. **157**(19): p. 54-9, 62, 64.

Lievre, A., D. Alley, and E.M. Crimmins, *Educational Differentials in Life Expectancy With Cognitive Impairment Among the*

Elderly in the United States. J Aging Health, 2008. **20**(4): p. 456-477.

Jaeggi, S.M., et al., *Improving fluid intelligence with training on working memory.* Proc Natl Acad Sci U S A, 2008. **105**(19): p. 6829-33.

Willis, S.L., et al., *Long-term effects of cognitive training on everyday functional outcomes in older adults.* JAMA, 2006. **296**(23): p. 2805-14.

References for section 4 – Optimum Sleep

Rechtschaffen, A., et al., *Sleep deprivation in the rat: X. Integration and discussion of the findings.* Sleep, 1989. **12**(1): p. 68-87.

Perceived insufficient rest or sleep--four states, 2006. MMWR Morb Mortal Wkly Rep, 2008. **57**(8): p. 200-3.

Ohayon, M.M., *Epidemiology of insomnia: what we know and what we still need to learn.* Sleep Med Rev, 2002. **6**(2): p. 97-111.

Kryger, M.H., T. Roth, and W.C. Dement, eds. *Principles and Practice of Sleep Medicine.* 4th ed. 2005, Elsevier Inc.: Philadelphia, PA.

Kuramoto, A.M., *Therapeutic benefits of Tai Chi exercise: research review.* Wmj, 2006. **105**(7): p. 42-6.

Ayas, N.T., et al., *A prospective study of self-reported sleep duration and incident diabetes in women.* Diabetes Care, 2003. **26**(2): p. 380-4.

Ayas, N.T., et al., *A prospective study of sleep duration and coronary heart disease in women.* Arch Intern Med, 2003. **163**(2): p. 205-9.

Meerlo, P., A. Sgoifo, and D. Suchecki, *Restricted and disrupted sleep: Effects on autonomic function, neuroendocrine stress systems and stress responsivity.* Sleep Med Rev, 2008. **12**(3): p. 197-210.

Zohar, D., et al., *The effects of sleep loss on medical residents' emotional reactions to work events: a cognitive-energy model.* Sleep, 2005. **28**(1): p. 47-54.

Breslau, N., et al., *Sleep disturbance and psychiatric disorders: a longitudinal epidemiological study of young adults.* Biol Psychiatry, 1996. **39**(6): p. 411-8.

334   *BrainFit For Life*

Weissman, M.M., et al., *The morbidity of insomnia uncomplicated by psychiatric disorders.* Gen Hosp Psychiatry, 1997. **19**(4): p. 245-50.

Medicine, I.o., *Sleep Disorders and Sleep Deprivation: An Unmet Public Health Problem.* 2006, Washington, DC: The National Academies Press.

Cole, M.G. and N. Dendukuri, *Risk factors for depression among elderly community subjects: a systematic review and meta-analysis.* Am J Psychiatry, 2003. **160**(6): p. 1147-56.

Ford, D.E. and D.B. Kamerow, *Epidemiologic study of sleep disturbances and psychiatric disorders. An opportunity for prevention?* Jama, 1989. **262**(11): p. 1479-84.

Czeisler, C.A., et al., *Chronotherapy: resetting the circadian clocks of patients with delayed sleep phase insomnia.* Sleep, 1981. **4**(1): p. 1-21.

Lack, L.C. and H.R. Wright, *Clinical management of delayed sleep phase disorder.* Behav Sleep Med, 2007. **5**(1): p. 57-76.

Chang, P.P., et al., *Insomnia in young men and subsequent depression. The Johns Hopkins Precursors Study.* Am J Epidemiol, 1997. **146**(2): p. 105-14.

Kessler, R.C., et al., *Lifetime and 12-month prevalence of DSM-III-R psychiatric disorders in the United States. Results from the National Comorbidity Survey.* Arch Gen Psychiatry, 1994. **51**(1): p. 8-19.

Knutson, K.L., et al., *The metabolic consequences of sleep deprivation.* Sleep Med Rev, 2007. **11**(3): p. 163-78.

Tasali, E., et al., *Slow-wave sleep and the risk of type 2 diabetes in humans.* Proc Natl Acad Sci U S A, 2008. **105**(3): p. 1044-9.

Kim, B., *Thyroid hormone as a determinant of energy expenditure and the basal metabolic rate.* Thyroid, 2008. **18**(2): p. 141-4.

Knutson, K.L., *Impact of sleep and sleep loss on glucose homeostasis and appetite regulation.* Sleep Med Clin, 2007. **2**(2): p. 187-197.

Spiegel, K., et al., *Sleep loss: a novel risk factor for insulin resistance and Type 2 diabetes.* J Appl Physiol, 2005. **99**(5): p. 2008-19.

Moisey, L.L., et al., *Caffeinated coffee consumption impairs blood glucose homeostasis in response to high and low glycemic index meals in healthy men.* Am J Clin Nutr, 2008. **87**(5): p. 1254-61.

Guzman-Marin, R., et al., *Suppression of hippocampal plasticity-related gene expression by sleep deprivation in rats.* J Physiol, 2006. **575**(Pt 3): p. 807-19.

Spiegel, K., J.F. Sheridan, and E. Van Cauter, *Effect of sleep deprivation on response to immunization.* Jama, 2002. **288**(12): p. 1471-2.

Banks, S. and D.F. Dinges, *Behavioral and physiological consequences of sleep restriction.* J Clin Sleep Med, 2007. **3**(5): p. 519-28.

Stickgold, R. and M.P. Walker, *Memory consolidation and reconsolidation: what is the role of sleep?* Trends Neurosci, 2005. **28**(8): p. 408-15.

Gais, S. and J. Born, *Declarative memory consolidation: mechanisms acting during human sleep.* Learn Mem, 2004. **11**(6): p. 679-85.

Balkin, T.J., et al., *Comparative utility of instruments for monitoring sleepiness-related performance decrements in the operational environment.* J Sleep Res, 2004. **13**(3): p. 219-27.

Belenky, G., et al., *Patterns of performance degradation and restoration during sleep restriction and subsequent recovery: a sleep dose-response study.* J Sleep Res, 2003. **12**(1): p. 1-12.

Millman, R.P., *Excessive sleepiness in adolescents and young adults: causes, consequences, and treatment strategies.* Pediatrics, 2005. **115**(6): p. 1774-86

INDEX

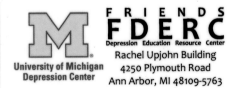

University of Michigan
Depression Center

F R I E N D S
FDERC
Depression Education Resource Center
Rachel Upjohn Building
4250 Plymouth Road
Ann Arbor, MI 48109-5763